Praise j

NO-BRAINER

Amber Gill is a kind, brilliant soul who cares about the health of others as much as she does the health of herself. Her heart is focused on getting people healthy and that is a gift to the world.

—**Jasmine Star**, Photographer and Business Strategist

Amber is brilliant. She has a unique gift for breaking down complex health topics in a way that's simple to understand and easy to apply, so that you can achieve optimum results! This book is full of warm, relatable stories and is such a fun read. After discovering Amber's surprisingly simple tips and tricks, you'll feel inspired to take control of your health for good in a meaningful, purposeful way.

—**Courtney M. Elmer**, Wellness Entrepreneur and Stress Expert

Reading this book is literally a NO-BRAINER! Not only does Amber give you all the simple, actionable tips and tools for becoming your best YOU, she does it in a way where you feel like you're talking to your BFF. She will make you laugh, feel better about yourself, and challenge you all at the same time. This is one you'll read, reread, and implement time and time again!

—**Jasmin Niemiec**, Business Coach

This girl rocked me! It's like she held a mirror up for me and just broke down all the things. She talked right to me, I laughed, I cried, and then I got started on my hacks. This book is a great addition to anyone's library, but especially if you've been feeling like you need someone to politely kick you in the rear in a good way, tell you all the hilarious and relatable stories and heartfelt ones, too, that created the desire to just be that 1% better! Amber reminds us over and over in this book just HOW to take that step, that 1% baby step to the life you crave and that we aren't alone in any it!

—Janel Gion, Website Design and Branding Photographer

The second I came across Amber, I immediately fell in love. I didn't even know her, but I wanted to be instant best friends. You know, the kind of best friend you need that calls you out, but holds your hair back when you over do it? AKA the friend who tells you like it is because she cares about you, but has 100% got your back when sh*t hits the fan.

If you want a book that's going to give you a pat on the back and reassure you that you're doing things right—this book is NOT for you. But if you're reading this right now, that tells me you're the type of person who wants to discover simple, small steps you can take every day to drastically improve your overall health and happiness. Don't walk, but RUN to grab this book off the shelf because it is seriously a no-brainer. Her advice is so practical and applicable that by page 30, I had already completely transformed the way I do life by tuning out the 99% of things that DON'T matter.

So do yourself a favor and pick up a copy, because you are just 1% a day away from living a life bigger and better than you could have ever imagined.

—Jilly Cedeño, Integrator and Launch Queen for James Wedmore

NO-BRAINER

NO-BRAINER

Simple Hacks To Increase Energy, Improve Productivity + Reduce Brain Fog

AMBER LANGLEY GILL

To the hubster.

The freaking love of my life.

With every wild idea I voice, you never question my ability to make it a reality. I will never understand just how fiercely you love me, but if it's just a sliver of how much I love you... then I am one blessed woman. Thank you for your unwavering support + confidence in my ability to fulfill this God-size dream in my heart.

CONTENTS

Introduction 7

Own Your Morning, Own Your Day! 11

    It Starts With Your Alarm Clock 12

    Put Your Armor On First 13

    Make Your Bed, Love 14

    Drink Some Water Before Caffeine 15

    A Lot More Gratta 15

    Feed Your Mind 17

    Move Your Body 18

Let's Not Diet 23

    Eat Your Greens 25

    Snack Wisely: Blueberries 27

    Snack Wisely: ER Food Stash 28

    Enjoy Healthy Fats 30

        Pumpkin Pancake Recipe 31

    Check Your Carbs 33

    Tying It All Together 34

        Protein 34

        Meal Prep 34

        Macronutrients/Caloric Intake 35

        Nourish Bowl Breakdown 36

Mom-Boss Up! 39

    Shift Your Focus 40

    Celebrate Wins 42

    Remove The Clutter 44

    Grab A Stress-Reducing Hobby 45

Give Yourself A Break 47

Make A "Ta-Da" List 48

Become A Nap Ninja 50

Move Your Tooshie 51

Evening Routine 53

Prep For Sleep During The Day 54

Get Your Game Face On! 54

    Do-It-Yourself Facial Mask Recipe 50

Hubster's Tip To Get Your ZZZ's 56

Turn Off Your Screens 56

Control Your Nightstand 57

Add Some Green To Your Bedroom 58

Be Good To The Skin You're In 61

What's On Your Pits? 61

The Best Beauty Trick 62

Wash Your Face, Love 64

Protect The Skin You Are In! 65

Take Care Of Your Feet 66

Consider Oil Pulling 67

Be Sweet To Your Skin 68

    Sugar Scrub Recipe 63

Transform Your Body And Mind With Movement 71

Find A Workout You Love 72

Schedule Movement Like A Boss 73

Work Out Even On Vacation 74

Up Your Workout Attire 75

Invest In Workout Socks 76

Set Out Your Clothes 77

Link Arms With A Fitness Buddy 78

Mix Up Your Workout Routine 79

Active Recovery..80
Add Some Foam Rolling...81
Fuel Your Body Well Post Workout...............................82

Your Biggest Weapon Is Within You.......................... 85

Celebrate Others...86
Laugh Hard And Laugh Often....................................87
Give Thanks..88
Lean In And Toss Out Perfection 89
Stay Present..90
Protect Your Inner Circle 92
Flip Your Script, Friend..93
Stop Flaking On You, Love 94
Speak Kindly To Yourself 95
Face Your Wall 97
Be You, Love 99

Final Words... 103

Further Book Recommendations 107

About the Author 101

INTRODUCTION

There is just something completely warped about dressing rooms, am I right? The lighting is set to make a gal look like an extra for the movie *Casper*, with pasty dry skin and dark blue circles under the eyes. Plus, where do they snag these mirrors that completely distort one's thighs to resemble bathroom mats. This can't be me, can it?

I stared at the reflection in the dim dressing room, holding a pair of jeans that didn't fit over my bathroom mat thighs. This woman was mimicking my moves but her hair was dry and thin with patchy, colorless skin. *Holy Toledo,* I thought. *This woman is me*—or at least the shell of who I was.

Somehow after our twins, the Gillies, made their arrival early at 27 weeks, and following the months in the NICU as well as multiple hospital stays afterwards, this was me. I was literally being held together by Jesus and a whole lot of dry shampoo and fueled by coffee.

Let's just say in that particular season of my life I felt like the term, "hot mess mom." And the reflection staring back at me would have to agree.

I remember just crying, hard. Not the pretty cry where tears magically stream down your face yet you still look put together. This was the other type of sobbing known as the ugly cry. You most likely have been there as well. The type of tears that pour from your bloodshot eyeballs, causing your nose to run and your face to sprout red splotches.

I was crying for so many reasons, it just hurt on the inside. I was crying because the hubster and I had spent almost a hundred days in the NICU with the Gillies fighting for their lives, and now my reflection looked like the ghost of Christmas past staring at me. How ridiculously horrible was I? The next day we were about to celebrate the Gillies turning one year old, and here I was sobbing hysterically while the hubster was trying to find me a pair of pants to cram all of me into.

Literally a hot mess.

It was in this blubbering moment of my life, the hubster opened the dressing room door with a stack of blue jeans of all different sizes. He looked at me and whispered to the Gillies who were nestled in their double stroller, "Look how beautiful your mama looks today."

Ugh. Insert another round of waterworks along with all the feelings in that particular moment that just came pouring out. How I knew my heart should be celebrating the twins' life—and it was—but I didn't recognize myself anymore. How I knew I should be grateful for that moment we'd fought so hard to get to, but....

The hubster placed a finger on my lips and gave me some tough love along with an idea.

I'll spare you all the mushy talk, but here's the main takeaway. He casually mentioned I should focus on simply doing one percent better each day—just one percent. Just not today and not tomorrow, but after the Gillies' birthday celebration.

For a person with a "Go BIG or Go HOME" attitude, this was hard for me to accept—both the delay in starting and the seemingly slow pace of one percent each day. But, I purchased a pair of bedazzled jeans and headed home with my head finally at peace. We celebrated the Gillies' first birthday and had professional photos taken to commemorate the day. I wore my bedazzled jeans, ate cake, and smiled so much that day my cheeks hurt.

Then the following day, I set my plan into action. The plan was to focus on being one percent better for one hundred consecutive days. Just one. If I focused on simply being one percent better each day, over time I would be doing 100 percent better than today. And how great would that feel, right? If you did the math, one percent each day for a hundred days would compound over time and total well better than 100 percent. But, let's not do math, shall we?

Throughout this book, you will see the habits I have developed over the past five years. The habits were born from trial and error. Some of them I picked up from attending live conferences like Brendon Burchard's High Performance Academy or Chalene Johnson's Market Impact Academy. Others are from books, which I tweaked to fit into my lifestyle. I'll make a list of my reading recommendations in the back of this book.

But here's the thing—these hacks aren't designed just to get you to fit into a pair of jeans. Nope. There's more to life than wearing bedazzled jeans with a certain number on the tag. The ghost staring back at me in the mirror wasn't just about a number. I had lost taking care of myself. I had lost who I was and had become a shell of the person I used to be.

This journey started as a way for me to climb back into her, a woman who was vibrant and energized. A woman whose skin was full of life and color. A woman who could form a complete sentence without having to rely on caffeine. A woman who carved out time for activities she found enjoyable and that breathed life into her. This idea of a hundred days of being one percent better was simply a way for me to start focusing on taking care of me. Shouldn't taking care of yourself be a no-brainer?

When reading this book, I just ask you do one thing—okay, maybe more than one thing.

+ Read the book as if a friend was sharing her favorite secrets with you, because I am.

+ Find one or two secrets that may work for you and explore them for a week.

+ Tweak a hack to fit into your life or allow it to inspire you to brainstorm other ideas.

+ Keep me posted on which hack has helped you in any way by taking a photo and tagging me on social (@mrsamberlgill on Instagram and Facebook) or shooting me a direct message on those platforms. I would absolutely love to hear from you. Unless it's not positive, then keep it to yourself. Ha.

+   Do not focus on doing everything all at once. Just focus on being one percent better *for you* today, that's it.

Now, let's find out which "no-brainer" hacks speak to you the best!

OWN YOUR MORNING, OWN YOUR DAY!

I can almost feel every reader's eyes roll upon reading this health hack—and I don't blame you. Not. One. Bit. Why? Because I totally understand where you are coming from. As a twin mama bear working as an emergency/critical care veterinarian, my mornings always felt rushed, crunched for time, and all I wanted was a chance to pee in peace for two lousy minutes.

Seriously.

How is it the hubster has *no* issues urinating with the door closed in silence—but as soon as my tooshie hits the porcelain queen's crown, the door springs open and I have 12,647 questions shouted at me. Once it startled me so much, I *almost* dropped my phone in the toilet.

Don't judge. We all watch YouTube videos on the toilet. You know you do, too.

Anywho. When my mornings would start later than I expected (a.k.a. hitting snooze eight times) and our twins, the Gillies, would rise shortly afterwards—my day would begin completely rushed. I would start the day feeling frazzled, disheveled, and not 100 percent on my A-game. Then by the time the day was done and my head hit the pillow, I'd begin thinking of how I didn't really show up as my best self for the Gillies, my clients, the hubster, or even myself. It wasn't until I took a *harsh* look at my life that I realized—how I started my day was crucial. Not just for the ability to pee in silence but to be the best version of me possible in every area of my life.

This means the best version of me as a mom, as a wife, as a coach, as a daughter, as a sister, as a friend, as *me*.

First thing you have to know about morning routines is the "best version" will look different to every single one of us. The best thing you can do is read the suggestions I provide, tweak them to your life, and take action. And if you are reading this saying, "Ugh, Amber. I work swing shift or overnights." Well, love. It still applies to you. Whenever you wake up and greet the day is when you need to *own your morning*. No matter what time the clock reads. Because I get it. I've lived it. Some of these tips I'm going to share, I discovered during my emergency/critical care residency—and my work hours were all over the place! And with that, let's dive deeper into my favorite hacks to *own your morning*.

It Starts With Your Alarm Clock

Have you ever noticed how easy it is to hit snooze on your cell phone's alarm? Incredibly easy. So simple, in fact, I am able to turn off my snooze at least eight times *before* fully waking up—and most of the time, I have no recollection of hitting the snooze *off*. The hubster, however, is fully aware just how many times I hit snooze and reminds me of this fact quite often.

He would wake up all grumpy pants, and I would feel stressed out for having overslept because I didn't hear my alarm. You can just imagine how awesome those morning conversations went. I do have to admit, the hubster is quite cute when he is grumpy. Yet I did have to figure out *how* exactly I would stop hitting snooze and start getting up in the morning. At least start getting up when my alarm would go off.

Insert the purchase of an old-school alarm clock.

Seriously. This move right here is simply genius. If this is the *only* health hack you take from this book, you are welcome. But it's not, so keep reading.

When I purchased an old-school alarm clock, a few things happened.

1. I stopped hitting snooze so many times because hitting the snooze on the alarm clock proved a wee bit more challenging.

2. I was able to fully turn *off* my phone and put it on airplane mode (sorry for folks who are on-call and need their phones to be on all the time, I feel you).

3. The hubster wasn't as cranky-pants face in the morning.

4. I didn't waste half an hour scrolling through social media first thing in the morning.

Did you read that last one? Read it again… I'll wait.

I didn't waste time first thing in the morning reading through social media, checking my emails or responding to text messages. I simply GOT UP! Do you have any idea how refreshing that is—and yet, so challenging this habit of mine was to break?

By using my phone as an alarm clock, I developed a habit of hitting snooze (on average four times). Then when I did wake up to turn off the alarm, I would scroll endlessly on social media catching up on what Sally did this morning while I was "snoozing," responding to Jane's email, or reading text messages, which would sometimes get me fired up.

The old school alarm clock was the best solution to help me conquer the snooze button—as silly as that sounds. And it doesn't have to be a top-notch alarm clock with all the bells and whistles. A $3 alarm clock from Walmart does just fine. Trust me.

Put Your Armor On First

When we start the day plugging into everything and everyone else around us, we automatically go into defense mode, and we can feel our bodies immediately tensing up. Why? Well, we start the day on *those* people's course, not the one God has set out for us personally. We start responding to *their* posts, to *their* questions, to *their* messages, and not to our own journey.

In a society where our phones are multi-tools, it is so easy to wake up (to your phone alarm) and automatically plug into the world around you. You may check out the news, start responding to messages, catch what Sally is wearing or even spot how far Jane ran this morning before *dawn*, is she crazy?!?

Once you dive into your phone, you immediately start responding—and your body hasn't even woken up yet! Seriously. Your feet haven't even touched the floor!

So, love. Here's the gist. Simply start the day with the phone *off*! You read that correctly, gorgeous. This means no social media, no emails, no returning messages, and no news surfing.

Starting my day with silence in focused prayer and listening to my own thoughts helps me put on my armor and start the day ready to *slay*!

Make Your Bed, Love

Did you know that supposedly, folks who make their beds are more productive? And now you are automatically pondering if your bed is currently made.

In a 2014 commencement speech at the University of Texas at Austin, Navy Admiral William McRaven said, "If you make your bed every morning, you will have accomplished the first task of the day. It will give you a small sense of pride and it will encourage you to do another task and another and another. By the end of the day, that one task completed will have turned into many tasks completed. Making your bed will also reinforce the fact that little things in life matter."

{BOOM}

Powerful words, love. The simple task of making your bed first thing in the morning has also been linked to increased productivity, lower stress levels, and improved mood—as well as better quality of sleep.

And it's not rocket science. Simply taking a beat to make your bed *first* thing is good for your health!

Another tip I have for you is to ditch the throw pillows. If throw pillows are your thing, then you do you, boo. However, I feel like throw pillows are the mom's version of an 8-year-old's stuffed animal collection. But hey, I didn't have a lot of stuffed animals on my bed growing up due to a *lice* outbreak in our tee-ball league. You are welcome for that memory.

Drink Some Water Before Caffeine

A year or two ago, starting the day off with water was *not* my strong suit. Sure, I had the water available (on the nightstand)! However, instead of *drinking* the water that was available, I would zombie walk down the hallway through the house to reach the bubbling coffee pot for some liquid caffeine.

Which means I would down a cup of coffee before properly hydrating myself. This habit would make me extremely grumpy, lethargic, and if not careful, suffering a headache an hour or two later. Why? Because I didn't truly understand the importance of proper hydration.

Studies have estimated 75 percent of Americans may suffer from chronic de-hydration. And you may be thinking, *I'm not dehydrated*, because you think of dehydration as vomiting, passing out, sticky mouth, crusty lips, and worse case scenario, death. However, dehydration covers a wide spectrum, and even mild dehydration can hinder our performance. How? Well, by decreasing our memory capabilities and increasing anxiety as well as fatigue!

Here's the health hack low-down. **Drink 8 ounces of water *first* thing in the morning**! Nowadays, I aim to drink at least 12 to 16 ounces of clean filtered water before my lips touch the coffee mug. For you, just make it simple and keep a bottle of water next to your bedside. This way, when you rise in the morning, it's ready to go! And you can sip your water while you do your own version of the zombie-walk to the coffee pot.

A Lot More Gratta

Since you are taking a beat in the morning to unplug from screens and spending a few moments in silence, I would love for you to reflect on the day before and the good that came to be, as well as how you would like this day to unfold.

When reflecting on the day before, simply replay yesterday's events. Did you grab groceries, bump into an old friend, get a letter in the mail that made you smile, stumble upon a hilarious quote, wear two socks without holes in the toes, progress in your handstand journey, spend a few minutes coloring with your littles, hear the words "I love you"?

There is always some good to recall, no matter how big or small.

Jot down at least three things that happened yesterday that made you smile. Just three experiences you enjoyed or appreciated. By doing this, you are shifting your focus towards gratitude.

This habit, I've discovered, works not only in your morning routine but also in other areas, such as work. I used to employ the "three gratta rule" as an emergency veterinarian! It was probably a wee bit annoying to my co-workers. Let's *not* ask them, okay? Anywho. The majority of patients coming into an emergency/critical care specialty clinic were super sick. But when a technician would walk back saying, "Oh, Langley, this furkid's kidney values are through the roof," I would say, "Okay, now give me three positives. No matter how big or small."

It never failed. The technician would immediately find three or more positive things to say about the furkid and we would move on—even if the situation was grim. Focusing on the positive shifted the energy in the room—or at least it did for me.

That's something I tell the Gillies, our twins, all the time (and let's be real, the hubster, too)—*a little less atta (a.k.a. attitude) and a bit more gratta (gratitude)!*

Moving on, love. After you take a beat to reflect on yesterday, casually glance at your list of what is planned for today. We all know life sometimes has other plans, but search for those moments you are grateful for in your upcoming agenda. Scoop them out and circle them.

Maybe you are able to bring your littles to school this morning, and you find joy in singing in the carpool lane with them. Are you meeting a friend for coffee, or did you pack your favorite salad to eat lunch in the park? No matter *what* it is, love, jot down where you can find joy today, and be grateful in that moment.

Feed Your Mind

You may be shocked to find out I'm not talking about nutrition. What I am talking about is the *noise* buzzing all around you. We live in a busy society where most of us have access to news, TV shows, YouTube videos, podcasts, and more, within arm's reach.

And to me, there's a lot of chatter out there—some good, but some not so good. The point is, we all *choose* what to feed our minds, simply by what we focus on. So, love, choose wisely.

Be aware of what you are plugging into, especially on commutes! For me, that's the perfect chance to *learn* via podcasts or audiobooks. One of my favorite mentors called her morning commute her "virtual classroom," and I love this analogy. Numerous podcasts are available to enhance your day, all with a click of a button. Now, you might be mumbling to yourself, "Amber, I don't have a commute!" Well, love, you can still plug into a podcast while doing daily tasks such as walking the furkids outside, putting on your makeup or brushing your teeth, taking a shower (just be careful to not get your phone wet), cooking dinner, or folding the endless piles of laundry!

There is always time to *feed your mind* well. Some of my favorite podcasts include:

+ Elevation Church with Pastor Steven Furtick

+ Marketing Made Easy with Amy Porterfield

+ RISE with Rachel Hollis

+ Doctor's Farmacy with Dr. Mark Hyman

+ Mind Your Business with James Wedmore

+ The Paleo Solution with Robb Wolf

+ ...the list could go on.

Now, you don't have to love these podcasts in particular, but it's a place to start. Find podcasts you love and start feeding your mind right!

Move Your Body

Moving your body is one thing I absolutely *love* to talk about. Why? Well, we all know there are numerous benefits to adding a wee bit of exercise (a.k.a. movement) to your day. But here's the thing, love, if I can get really personal with you for a moment.

See, I'm the youngest of three girls, and my two older sisters were diagnosed with a form of muscular dystrophy when I was quite young. Growing up, I always appreciated the ability I had to move my body in whatever way I chose—to run, bend, strengthen, dance, flex.

We were built to *move* and not be stagnant. Now, sometimes, you can't move due to injury or medical condition. Trust me, I get it. Just listen to *your* body, love, and do what you can for a wee bit.

When I say "wee bit," I really mean it. Just 20 minutes! That's literally less than 2 percent of your day. You are worth more than 2 percent of your day, no?

Now. One reason I love working out first thing in the morning is because it may help reduce brain fog and allows you to be more productive throughout the day, by at least 20 percent! HELLO!

Seriously, that's the number I read—20 percent more productive! Can you *imagine* how productive you will be? Plus, working out gives you endorphins, which send happy-positive vibes to your brain, meaning your mood will drastically improve!

{Channeling my inner Elle Woods: Happy people just don't shoot their husbands, they just don't!}

The final reason I love to bust a sweat (just 20 minutes) first thing in the morning is because life happens and you never know when you will be able to squeeze in a workout if you don't just *do it*! And if I'm being 100 percent real with you, if I wait to work out when our twins (the Gillies) go to bed, I will *not* be working out that day. It's just the truth. I know myself.

Plus, who likes to have something hanging over their head during the day? Am I right? The longer you put it off, the more you will dread it and the more miserable you will be throughout the day. I have discovered this from years of procrastinating my workout. Just get a 20-minute workout *first* thing in the morning and be proud of yourself for taking time for you and your health.

NOTE: A 20-minute workout doesn't have to be a crossfit-style balls-out sweat fest (if that's your thing—good on ya!). Just *move* your body. Go for a walk with the pup, dance to Taylor Swift in your living room, take an online workout class, or head to the gym. Just do something that makes you smile and gets your blood pumping. More on fitness later, love. I promise!

Whew! As I mentioned before, it's all about figuring out what works for you—tweaking bits and taking action. So, I would love for you to take a beat and jot down what the *perfect* start to your morning looks like. (But make it realistic, I mean, the *perfect* start to my day would be to wake up and get a deep tissue massage then hop in the steam room for 10 minutes before sitting down to a chef-prepared breakfast of lobster Benedict, am I right?) Picture your (reasonable) perfect morning and make it happen. What would it look like for you?

Break It Down

Sometimes, you just want to see it laid out, don't you? I get it, so here's the flow of how I set myself up to *own my morning*. Just hear me on this: do what works best for *you*. We are all in different seasons and situations in life. Take one hack at a time, tweak it to your liking, and give yourself space, knowing these new habits *will* take time.

+ **Alarm clock:** Opt for an old-school alarm clock to wake you up in the morning instead of your phone.

+ **Make your bed:** Enough said, right? Even when the hubster is still sleeping and I get up for the day, I will make my side of the bed. True story.

+ **Journal:** I absolutely love taking a beat to spend in gratitude *first* thing in the morning. A journal I have enjoyed is *Let That Sh*t Go* by Monica Sweeney. I also love spending time in a devotional called *Jesus Calling* by Sarah Young. Journaling time is also when I drink my morning coffee—not going to lie. It's delicious and it makes me chuckle thinking I'm having "coffee with Jesus."

+ **Podcasts:** When I'm getting ready for the day (brushing teeth/ washing face), a podcast is playing so I can soak up as much knowledge as possible. I recommend creating a list of podcast episodes you want to listen to, so you never waste time in the morning searching for a good one.

+ **Drinking water:** Each night, I place a 24-ounce water bottle on the nightstand. I drink about half of the water before I go to bed and the rest of the water when I wake up in the morning. My bottle of choice is an army green Yeti Tumbler.

+ **Move the tooshie:** Working out is something I don't enjoy doing until it's over. I do love the feeling of completing a session, no matter how intense it was. It's best to do something you enjoy and to schedule it into your morning routine. For me, I love to sneak in a morning run or take part in an at-home workout session. You do you, boo.

Take Action, Love

Break out your phone and set the timer for 10 minutes, no more, and then turn it on airplane mode. In the next 10 minutes, you are going to brainstorm what your perfect start to the morning will look like. There's no right or wrong answer; it may look like mine, it may not, and that's beautiful. Just make it realistic, and give yourself space to form this habit over time.

LET'S NOT DIET

I have to be completely real with you.

As I sit here writing my nutritional hacks, I'm battling a ginormous craving for chips and salsa. No lie. I even just sent my bestie a voice text stating how badly I was craving the salty goodness *while* writing this chapter. She thought I should mention this to you… so there. Just keeping things real. And no, I didn't cave.

Anywho. Let's get back to the topic—diet. Ugh! Seriously, this word makes my skin crawl. It's kinda like the word "moist." Am I right? Grossness! Those are the two words I dislike most in the English language. I once read a blog post that suggested we simply switch the letters of DIET to EDIT—and focus on *editing* what we eat.

Genius! I truly wish I could remember who wrote the article because I like to give credit where credit is due—and this idea is pure gold. Instead of dieting, just *edit* what you eat—and do so in a way that not only nourishes your body, but also brings you joy.

I'm not saying it's okay to down a bag of Cheetos for dinner because licking slabs of artificial cheese powder off your fingers brings you complete joy. I'm saying find a style of eating that is good for your body *and* makes you happy. The "happy" part is necessary in order to stick with it long-term.

For me, I'm all about focusing on unprocessed or unpackaged foods that contain *real* ingredients to nourish my body. And yes, this does mean all four food groups! Yikes! I'm talking about carbohydrates here, love!

My name is Amber and I eat carbs!

There, I said it. Now, if we are being completely transparent, I'll also say this. I haven't always had a healthy relationship with food. It's true. I grew up in the Deep South where second helpings were *always* a thing, and Grandma Broussard didn't let you leave her house without a belly full of home cooking. In high school and early years of college, I had such a negative relationship with food that if it hadn't been for the hubster (who was my best friend at the time) speaking to me about my overall health, things could have turned out pretty bad.

I'll even admit to trying almost every DIET out there—paleo, vegan, keto, vegetarian, South Beach, Atkins, and even my hideous attempt of trying the lemon juice and cayenne only diet (which I strongly do not recommend).

What I do recommend is listening to your body as well as your primary care physician to discover which nutritional journey is right for you. I am not a nutritionist. I am not a registered dietitian. I am not a human medical doctor. I am human and I am a doctor; however, I was trained in treating and diagnosing species other than humans. I am a veterinarian.

So why am I sharing all this with you? Because when our twins, the Gillies, were born, I realized I needed to focus on optimal brain health for one child, and gut health for the other. The only thing I had any control over while they were in the Neonatal Intensive Care Unit was their nutrition (hello, breastfeeding warrior). I knew focusing on *my* nutrition would help the Gillies with their health, and this opened my eyes entirely to the world of nutrition.

I also think we complicate things way too much. For example, you *know* eating a bag of cheesy puffs at 2 a.m. is not a healthy choice. Right? You do know this? Not that I don't love cheesy puffs. I do! It was one of the favorite snacks my grandma used to give me after school. But I do know they aren't a healthy choice (especially the quantity I can put down).

If you are thinking, *Well,* you *believe nutrition is simple, Amber, but* how *is it simple*? Let me share with you this brilliant saying I once heard:

"If it came from a plant or ate a plant, it's okay. If it was *made* in a plant (i.e., packaged/processed), think twice."

See. Brilliant and so simple.

But *why* should you care? Well, here's a ridiculously scary prediction I read recently, which was sourced by the American Academy of Neurology: By the year 2050, approximately 14 million people in the United States will have Alzheimer's disease.[1] And to help you wrap your gorgeous brain around this—that's roughly the entire current population of New York City, Los Angeles, and Chicago combined.

What the what?!?

Sobering, right? So let's get to it. Just know after I share with you my hacks on how to load your plate for optimal brain and gut health, you'll also receive some pointers to help you *after* your plate is loaded. Baazinga!

Eat Your Greens

Our twins have a favorite saying that channels their inner Popeye: "I'm strong to the finish, 'cause me eat me spinach." And that's how we are kicking off our nutritional health hacks: *eat your greens*! The book *The Better Brain Solution* mentions eating a cup of green leafy vegetables every day will make you, on average, 11 years physiologically younger than someone who doesn't!

{Did you hear that... someone just shut the front door.}

Some of my go-to leafy greens include spinach, kale, brussels, swiss chard, dandelion greens, and more. Personally, I like to sneak spinach into smoothies, toss them into scrambled eggs, or serve as a big sass salad with a droopy egg on top. Simply delicious.

Another cool factoid about leafy greens is they are loaded with fiber, vitamin K, folate, potassium, antioxidants, anti-inflammatory properties, and so

---

1   https://www.alzinfo.org/articles/alzheimers-cases-triple-2050/

much more. And your cells will be physiologically younger if you eat leafy greens daily, so it's good for your heart, brain, and bones.

Need some ideas on how to get your greens in each day? I got your back. Here you go:

+ **Juice 'em:** I'm always a fan of juicing leafy greens yourself rather than purchasing in a bottle from a store. If you can't juice them at home, find a local juicery that can make you a fresh juice filled with leafy greens, ginger root, a wee bit of lemon, and maybe an apple.

+ **Breakfast:** Seriously, we need to get our minds thinking breakfast isn't just about sugary carbs and flip the switch to adding leafy greens to our plates. Try big salads for breakfast, serve sautéed greens on the side with eggs, or chop them up for omelettes!

+ **Smoothies:** I absolutely love adding frozen spinach leaves to my smoothies. To answer the questions: No, you cannot taste the frozen spinach leaves. Yes, frozen spinach leaves are the best because you reduce waste *and* you won't need to use as many ice cubes. You are welcome.

+ **Wraps:** Consider wrapping your sandwiches or burgers with Bibb lettuce instead of bread. You still get the flavor, yet lettuce wraps are packed with more powerful nutrients!

+ **Greens powder:** This is my least favorite way to consume greens because, well, it tastes like I'm licking a lawn mower, which I have never actually done but suspect that's what it would taste like. The hubster, however, loves drinking a green powder (mixed with water). Each time he chugs down a glass, he looks at me with such pride of accomplishment and says, "11 years younger."

+ **Salads:** I know this one is pretty easy; you had to know it was coming. Yet, when you are planning your meals, don't feel discouraged to serve "just a salad." Salads can be delicious, hearty, and fun! Get creative. Recreate salads from your favorite restaurant. Ask if you can purchase some of their homemade salad dressing. (I have done this before!) Just make sure when you build a salad that you add at least one to two handfuls of leafy greens (not iceberg lettuce) to the bowl.

Snack Wisely: Blueberries

Blueberries are one of my favorite snacks, and they remind me of the hubster. His side of the family used to operate a blueberry farm, and I got pretty spoiled. Each summer, we enjoyed stacks of gallon Ziploc® bags packed full of freshly picked blueberries for the taking. Delicious!

And now, whenever we head out to a farmer's market, fresh berries are always a must (along with cut flowers). It just reminds me of a time when we were first dating, back in college, getting free food (like the blueberries) from family members who felt pity for us broke students. His family would send me home with blueberries, and my folks would send me home with a case of tuna fish (because my dad had a Sam's Club card)! Ha!

Fish + blueberries = not a good combo; I'm not recommending it here. {Insert: gross face.}

Anywho. Blueberries are little powerhouses, check it:

+ Antioxidant properties
+ Protect against cognitive decline
+ May help lower cholesterol
+ May help improve memory, concentration, and coordination
+ Loaded with vitamin C
+ May help prevent heart disease!

There are so many reasons I love snacking on blueberries and why they are my go-to snack food. Just always try to opt for local and organic blueberries if you can, and don't pair them with canned tuna fish.

How do I like my blueberries? Here are some ideas:

+ Topped with melted almond butter atop fresh homemade pancakes (pumpkin pancakes are the best)

+ Tossed in a salad with leafy greens, roasted walnuts and a smidge of feta cheese

+ Blended into a smoothie for an afternoon brain boost

+ Dipped in Greek yogurt then placed in the freezer for a quick cool snack

Can you just *see* how much I love blueberries? Now let's talk about my other favorite smart snack: an ER food stash.

Snack Wisely: ER Food Stash

ER FOOD STASH: emergency food stash (*noun*).

An ER food stash is what I call a variety of healthy snacks you keep on person, in vehicle or office desk, where you can grab with ease to ward off food cravings and stick to your health goals.

This concept was developed after a *hangry* event that led to this mama bear cursing herself out after stopping at Sonic for a chicken wrap and Diet Coke—please, no judgement. It's all about knowing better in order to do better, right?

Nowadays, our emergency food stash includes the following:

+ Mason jar filled with fresh blueberries (no lie)

+ Mason jar filled with cashews (for our little man)

+ Mason jar filled with pistachios (for our little miss)

+ Beef jerky (for the hubster)

+ Collection of nutritional bars (Larabar, Protein Puck, RXBAR)

+ Mason jar filled with homemade mix (dried cranberries, pumpkin seeds, walnuts, and dark chocolate)

Here's the thing though, love. Besides the fresh blueberries (and sometimes strawberries, in season), which I pack and snack the same day, the rest of the ER food stash remains in the vehicle at all times. Why? Because life gets complicated and sometimes we are rushing out the door to make it to this or that appointment. The last thing I need to do before an errand is worry about snacks for road trips. So, I keep an ER food stash in the vehicle for, well, emergencies.

I will also note that in the past, I have stashed candies known as fireballs. Not for the Gillies, but for myself. Fireball candies were my staple study treat in veterinary school because I read somewhere that cinnamon helps the brain retain information. Hello, any extra boost I could get in veterinary school, the better. However, I feel these candies could be bad for your teeth as well as the lining of the gut. I have no scientific proof; these are just my suspicions from experience (although, my penchant for these candies was pretty high). Anywho. I stopped keeping them in the vehicle as one day I was driving the Gillies to yet another appointment when I started *choking* on a fireball.

I ended up pulling over to the side of the road to catch my breath. It was in that moment, I decided to never pop another fireball again—unless the hubster was nearby to perform the Heimlich procedure. Can you just imagine the obituary: twin mom passed away today due to fireball consumption!

Your takeway: Build your own ER food stash to prevent future poor food choices and to minimize the appearance of the *hangry* monster; consider adding blueberries to your grocery list, and rethink hard candies when driving alone or with kids.

Enjoy Healthy Fats

Sometimes following the nutritional trends feels sorta like whiplash, right? Fats are good for you. Fats are bad. Fats make you fat. Opt for low-fat. Opt for fat-free. Yikes!

It's a wee bit overwhelming, but I'll share with you one tidbit. Don't be scared of *healthy* fats! You will not get fat by simply eating fat; there are a whole lot of other things that can cause weight gain. Deep breath.

In our house, we munch on healthy fats, moderate amounts of clean protein sources, and small portions of carbohydrates, which we snag from mostly vegetables and some fruits. However, I am *still* craving chips and salsa. No lie.

Here's the thing, though. You do you, boo. If noshing an occasional basket of chips does not compromise your personal health or convictions, then by all means, set your own limits. I'm just sharing what works for my family and the brains/guts in our house. We've personally learned to cut out certain foods altogether because our bodies operate better without them. Your body might be different. Just follow the general rule of eating mostly clean choices, and you'll be way better off than someone who inhales a party-size bag of Cheetos every night.

Moving on. Healthy fats, why? Well, besides helping you feel full longer (thereby preventing overeating) and tasting good, fats are also good for your immune system! Woot woot!

If you need help in knowing *what* to choose, here are some of my faves:

+ Fresh avocado
+ Handful of nuts (walnuts, almonds, macadamias, pistachios, barukas)
+ Pasture-raised eggs (not fed a vegetarian diet)
+ Grass-fed and grass-finished beef/bison
+ Fatty wild-caught fish
+ Coconut oil
+ Dark chocolate (we will touch on this soon)

Here's the thing though, when I say *nuts*—I'm NOT talking about peanuts. Fun fact: Peanuts are technically not nuts, but legumes. I know—"nut" is in the name, but it's not a nut. Neither is a coconut. Yikes!

Anywho. Nuts are freaking amazing, and I think they get a bad rap for being so fatty; however, when you think about it, your gorgeous brain is made up of nearly 60 percent fat! Hello.

This means you need a good dose of dietary fat to nourish your brain. *The Better Brain Solution* states that "nuts are one of the most brain-nourishing choices you can make."

{BOOM}

Just consider reaching for nuts as a healthy snack alternative. One of my favorite nuts is barukas, which are loaded with fats, protein, fiber, and magnesium. Plus, they taste like roasted peanuts (and I scored on Amazon). So good.

And as I mentioned earlier, one of my favorite treats is to top off a pile of fresh pumpkin pancakes with almond butter and a bonus of blueberries. Ugh, so delicious. Here is my pumpkin pancake recipe so you can try them yourself.

Pumpkin Pancake Recipe

Ingredients

+ ½ cup of pumpkin
+ ⅓ cup of maple syrup
+ 4 eggs, whisked
+ ¼ cup of almond flour
+ 4 tbsp of coconut oil, melted
+ 1 tsp of baking soda
+ 1 tbsp of baking powder
+ 1 tsp of cinnamon
+ 1 tsp of ginger
+ 1 tbsp of pumpkin spice
+ Dash of himalayan pink salt

Now What?

1. Using a griddle or skillet, lightly grease and set the temperature at 300F degrees or medium heat.

2. Melt the coconut oil in a glass measuring bowl then add the eggs to the melted oil and whisk away.

3. Add the pumpkin to the egg/oil mixture and blend, then add the maple syrup and, you guessed it, blend again.

4. Now, add all the dry ingredients and spices to the pumpkin mixture. Stir until the batter is fully blended.

5. Once the griddle or skillet is warm and ready, spoon out a wee bit of the mixture on the hot surface.

6. When you see bubbles forming on the pumpkin mixture, gently flip over and cook the other side.

7. Remove from heat and set aside while continuing to repeat steps 5-7 until all the pancakes are made.

Check Your Carbs

When diving deep into what works with *my* gut, I stumbled upon something known as "carb cycling." It's basically a fancy way of saying you focus on *when* you eat your carbohydrates.

My gut does best when I save my carbohydrates (the slow or complex carbs) for the evening meal. Why, exactly? Well, I read somewhere that it can improve melatonin production for a better night's sleep and help with regulating hormones.

So, basically, I sleep better and my hormones are in check.

Winner-winner-sweet taters with my dinner.

What are some slow carb options? Some of my favorites include:

+ Colorful and sweet taters
+ Pumpkin and winter squashes
+ Quinoa and beets
+ Carrots
+ Jerusalem artichokes

Just to name a few. If I'm being completely honest, I do love me some sweet potatoes. My mom used to say that when I was a baby the doctor asked her to stop feeding me so many yams and sweet potatoes because my skin was actually turning orange! Yikes!

Some ways I love to incorporate these slow carbs is by peeling and blending in a food processor until they are as small as a grain of rice, then sautéeing in a skillet with a wee bit of ghee. So good. In our house, we also replaced noodles with spaghetti squash and switched out rice for quinoa! It's all about baby steps. Another truth-sharing moment: we still have medium grain rice with our gumbo. It's the Cajun in me; I cannot and will not substitute *rice* in gumbo. It's not natural.

Takeaway: Remember, saving slow carbs for dinner is how *I* do carbs. You do *you*, boo—which means listen to your body and decide for yourself how it responds to "checking your carbs." Then choose what works best for you!

Tying It All Together

So far we've talked about how to build an ER stash to reduce the "hangry monster," plus I shared why I focus on leafy greens, healthy fats, and healthy carbohydrates. I didn't dive into protein sources, how to meal prep, or knowing your macronutrients/caloric intake. Here's why:

Protein

Some folks are vegan, vegetarian, or keto. I have tried all three and trust me, my gut needs me to *not* be any of them. My gut, not yours. The type of protein I reach for includes wild-caught seafood, grass-fed beef/bison, and pasture-raised eggs. I'm not a huge fan of poultry or pork. That's just my preference. You do you, boo. (I'm going to say that a lot, are you catching on?)

Meal Prep

I have experience coaching folks on how to prepare meals, and I even sell a collection of menus with grocery lists and prep tips on my website. However, meal prepping is not for everyone, and truth be told, I don't personally enjoy it all that much. There's something about seeing stacks of pre-prepared Tupperware in my fridge that sets me on edge. So since it's not my personal passion, I'm not going to emphasize meal planning here.

Macronutrients/Caloric Intake

Personally I discovered I needed to stop focusing so much on numbers and shift my attention instead to the *types* of foods I eat. Do you focus intently on calories? Do you get overwhelmed with macronutrient ratios? How much fat? How many carbs? Ugh. Do I need more protein?

It's all too overwhelming and, quite honestly, a slippery slope for me. Because once I start tracking numbers, that's *all* I think about, and my attitude towards food becomes aggressive instead of realizing food is a gift to my body. Food gives us the ability to heal and nourish! How wonderful is that?

One of the goals I set for myself is to shift my focus away from counting calories and macronutrients (eeek!) and simply look at my plate. Is it loaded down with leafy greens? A clean protein source? Healthy fats?

Basically—*real ingredients.*

One solution I have discovered is nourish bowls, which are exactly what the name implies—a bowl full of nourishing ingredients. This recipe can be a mixture of foods you enjoy. Here is the backbone to creating your own nourish bowl.

"When you start eating food without labels, you no longer need to count calories."

–Amanda Kraft

Nourish Bowl Breakdown

+ Leafy greens (majority): kale, arugula, spinach, dandelion greens, mustard greens, collards, romaine, Swiss chard

+ Vegetables (or fruits): asparagus, beets, carrots, cucumbers, onions, radishes, tomatoes, blueberries, pears, bananas

+ Clean protein source: grass-fed beef, chicken, pasture-raised eggs, shrimp, salmon, protein powder, tofu, hemp seeds, quinoa—although I use this as a carb source!

+ Carbohydrates: gluten-free oats, quinoa, sweet potato, squash, rice noodles, wild rice, couscous

+ Healthy fats: avocado, olives, almonds, pumpkin seeds, sesame seeds, coconut oil, EVOO

Other ingredients you can add to the mixture that I love are: sauerkraut (gut health benefits), certain types of superfood powders (i.e., cacao, matcha, spirulina), fresh herbs for additional flavor and health benefits, as well as spices such as turmeric or cinnamon!

Okay. Now let's build ourselves a nourish bowl, love.

1. Start with a handful of leafy greens. I like to keep a bunch of leafy greens washed and chopped in an airtight container so I can simply grab and go quickly.

2. Reach for fresh vegetables in a variety of colors! Our Gillies are huge asparagus fans, so in order to make sure they get their greens, mama has become an asparagus fan, too. You feel me? It's all in the greater good, loves… the greater good.

3. Add some carbohydrates. For me, it's typically sweet potatoes or quinoa. The Gillies aren't exactly quinoa enthusiasts; however, someone once told me a child needs to be introduced to a food *nine* times or more before they will actually try it. Nine times!?! Is this true? Well, I haven't done any official research into the matter. Just speaking

from personal experience, it takes ninety-nine times for my son to cave. That may or may not be an exaggeration.

4. Include a clean protein source. One of my favorites is sunny-side-up eggs because the yolk acts as a "dressing," making the bowl super yummy (to me!). One tip: Opt for pasture-raised eggs if you can, because this means the chickens have access to natural food sources like bugs and grubs, plus they spend their days not cooped up inside but enjoying the sunshine.

5. Finally, add healthy fats. I'm typically reaching for an avocado, which we call "nature's butter" in our household because it's full of good healthy fats, which your brain absolutely loves, and the creamy texture is simply delicious.

And that's how to tie it all together in the form of a nourish bowl. Take a beat to think of how you could make your own bowl. What would it look like? What are some healthy fats you could use? Your favorite clean protein source? Which leafy greens would you start with? Be creative. One of our favorites is a hamburger bowl, which combines a homemade meatball, leafy greens, broccoli and sweet potatoes topped with mashed avocado! Ugh, so delicious—let's all have it for dinner tonight!

 Nourish bowls don't technically have to be *bowls*. Your "bowl" can mean a smoothie with vegan protein powder and a side salad or cup of soup. However, I like the term "nourish bowls" because it sounds like a bowl of comfort filled with gut-nourishing foods. Comfy, healthy, and delicious!

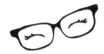

MOM-BOSS UP!

This hack may sting a wee bit because sometimes, like the saying goes, "the truth hurts." A while back a mentor of mine casually said something that spoke to me. He said:

"When working with people, I always ask—if you were healthy, who would it benefit?"

Right. Did that question feel like a sucker punch in the gut? But ask yourself, IF you took care of yourself—really took care of YOU and changed your habits—who would that help?!?

{Gut check}

For me, it was abundantly clear who would benefit besides myself. The Gillies, our twins, would definitely benefit from a mom with clean, positive energy. A mom with a mind that was more alert and engaging. Plus, my attitude would most likely be more inspiring and encouraging.

Next would be the hubster, who would benefit from a wife who felt strong and confident in her skin. He would have a wife who was more engaging in conversation and also a wee bit more present and focused, especially in discussions regarding budgets.

Last but not least, my clients would benefit. This includes both furkids and humans. As a veterinarian or a coach, I would be more mentally aware and attentive. I would be up on the latest trends and treatments plus be energized, encouraging, and motivating.

Many others would benefit if I simply took time to really take care of me.

Now comes the question most folks would ask (heck, I did)—but what does that look like, exactly? How do you take care of yourself?

Well. This chapter is all about how I "mom-boss UP" by taking care of me without getting overwhelmed with all the day-to-day tasks.

If you aren't a mom, no worries, love. These hacks will still apply to you! If you are a mom but don't have a business, no worries either. These hacks will still help you out. It's all about taking care of you.

Before we dive in, I'll share with you a few little tweaks in my daily life that actually helped me mom-boss UP! Maybe there's one you already do or may consider implementing yourself. Here goes:

1. Rising up a wee bit early to get my morning workout in

2. Choosing reading over watching a TV show

3. Opting for water over diet soda/energy drinks

4. Fueling my plate with gut-healing foods

5. Owning my business hours and my family time, scheduling my evening routine and holding true to it

6. Purchasing fresh flowers to spruce up the house

7. Epsom salt baths... enough said

Remember as you read through this chapter, the smallest things can make the biggest impact, love. So make sure to take care of YOU, and let me ask you the same question my mentor asked me. Who would benefit if YOU were truly taking care of YOU? Take a beat to think before reading on.

Shift Your Focus

Have you ever heard the saying, "You attract what you think about"? Let me share with you this little story about the time I decided to purchase a new vehicle.

The hubster and I were newly married, living in northern Pennsylvania and driving a beat up old pickup truck—in the winter months. The truck was nearly 13 years old and had survived multiple cross-country trips and two hurricanes. This truck had also succumbed to two robberies, which resulted in a driver's side door handle that was basically non-existent. The radio didn't work, the windshield wipers were temperamental, and the A/C had given up long ago when we were living in the South. Anywho. On that beautiful icy day, I exited our building's parking lot to embark on my two-mile commute to work, when the truck's brakes decided *not* to work AT ALL. I was basically Flintstoning the brake pedal and flipping the truck into neutral as I coasted into a snowbank. Our day ended with a trip to the nearby Jeep dealership.

The funny thing was, I really hadn't seen a lot of Jeeps on the streets. I was worried Jeeps wouldn't be safe on the icy mountains of Pennsylvania. This is when something strange happened over the course of the following two weeks. All of a sudden I saw Jeeps on the roads. It felt like everyone in the Poconos area was out celebrating their purchase of a new Jeep. However, this wasn't the case. My mind was just *attracting* Jeeps to its attention, which means I was becoming more aware of Jeeps around me.

I am pretty sure there wasn't an influx of Jeep purchases, but just a matter of me becoming more aware. This brings me to my mom-boss UP hack for you: manage your focus. Think of your mind like a camera. What you focus on is what's captured, right? It's what is important in that moment. So focus on the *good* things in your life, and attract more of those moments. When life gets dark or you find yourself in a negative place, develop from those moments, and grow. And when things don't work out, just take another shot. Life is too short, so manage your focus.

Tips that help me manage my focus:

+ If a negative outcome occurs, I allow myself five minutes to pout, vent, or get angry. I set a timer on the phone and lash out all the feels. When the timer goes off, I write down how I can learn from this moment and move on. Don't dwell.

+ Spend time each morning in a state of gratitude with a journal. I tend to jot down three things I am grateful for. There's no science behind the number three; it just happens to be my favorite number. Sometimes, my words of gratitude are intense and deep. Other times, I'm channeling my inner eighth grade self with my lack of maturity. It is all good. Just jot down three things you are grateful for in that moment.

+ Before I lay my head down to sleep at night, I re-read those three blessings. There's something magical about going to bed with a grateful heart.

Celebrate Wins

When is the last time you celebrated an accomplishment? Hmm, I am guessing a loooonngggg time ago. When mapping out a huge goal—whether that's a fitness goal, weight loss goal, business venture, family goal, etc.—we sometimes forget to celebrate milestones. So, I am giving you permission to celebrate the wins along the way.

This approach helped me drop 30 pounds. But first, let me pump the brakes and say this. I lost those 30 pounds *after* pregnancy and a *year* after the Gillies came home from the NICU. It didn't happen overnight, nor did it happen in a year. It was many months until I realized that if I continued to focus on the *end game* (i.e., losing 30 pounds), I would constantly be riding this rollercoaster.

So. I broke down my goal into other milestones, such as: Was my nutrition spot-on all week? Did I drink enough water in a day? How were my pants fitting? Did I work out four times that week, etc.? The end goal was the same—to have more energy to keep up with the growing twins and to get out of my pregnancy jeans (no judgement, I wore mine far too long after the babies were born). However, I also stayed focused on how I would celebrate these milestones.

Some of these treats included:

+ A full body massage
+ A new facial mask I had been eyeing
+ An avocado T-shirt
+ A pair of J.Crew shorts to show off my hard work
+ A night to binge-watch my favorite TV series

Now. Whatever goal you have set for yourself, I would love for you to take a beat and celebrate the small wins with something you find rewarding! Just be cautious that these celebrations don't set you back. (For example, don't binge eat Ben & Jerry's when you are trying to shed some poundage, or if your goal is to launch a brand new course, blowing off a week to binge-watch The Bachelor may not be conducive to the goal.)

If you need some ideas to help celebrate your small wins along the way, here's ya go:

+ Seriously, full body massage
+ Renting a bike to explore your city
+ Meeting up with a friend for coffee and celebrating
+ Grabbing a book you have been eyeing and cuddling up on the couch
+ Catching a concert near you
+ Signing up for a new class and falling in love with a new hobby
+ An Epsom salt bath with some music playing quietly nearby

Take some time to brain dump ways you can celebrate your small wins. Just make sure you aren't celebrating with *tasks* on your "to-do" list and are actually taking a moment to cherish your success, no matter how small.

Remove The Clutter

In 2006, I visited South Africa for a wildlife conservation internship, which was brilliant and contains a whole bag of stories; however, I'll keep it to the point of this book. While on this trip, I bought a gorgeous handmade bowl. It was decorated with giraffes painted in an array of ambers, blacks, and whites. The bowl *was* freaking gorgeous.

Did you catch the past tense there?

On my travels back to the States, the bowl broke. I'm not talking about one simple crack. This bowl shattered into a thousand pieces. However, over the years, I attempted to glue and mold the bowl back together. As luck would have it, the bowl just wouldn't stay together and has ended up becoming more glue than actual bowl.

Despite all this, I have packed this bowl with me for over 12 years. Twelve years, people!?! It has traveled to seven different states and lived (in pieces) in eight different homes, wrapped in a towel with the promise to put it back together one day.

However, with our latest move across the country, I glanced over all the things I needed to pack and admitted some items were broken, missing a piece, or even lopsided. This made me realize, even though I cherished these items and the memories they held, I didn't love how these items made me *feel*—because they reminded me I wasn't taking time to repair them.

So. I chucked the lot of them.

I held each item in my hands and recalled the memories they gave me, then tossed them into a garbage bag. Do you know what I felt afterwards? Immediate release.

The feeling of letting things go and not being dragged down with hopes of fixing one day led me to look around at other items that were simply cluttering my life. Loose leaf papers, receipts from a luncheon months ago, old calendars, and clothes I couldn't (or shouldn't) wear. Hello, neon green bell bottoms, I'm looking at you! Don't ask.

I'd love for you to take a beat and look around. Are you clinging to certain items in hopes of one day restoring them? Have you been carrying around a broken giraffe bowl—or neon green bell bottoms—for twelve years?

If the memories are too intense to depart with the broken item, then by all means fix it! But if you can, remove the clutter and give yourself the release.

Here's a hack that helped me declutter:

+ Set a day to go through one room at a time.

+ In each room, mark items: toss, give away, or keep.

+ If you aren't planning on fixing an item but are having trouble parting with it, take a photo of the item before tossing. Store photos in a box to glance at when you want to recall those memories.

Grab A Stress-Reducing Hobby

When the Gillies were just one year old and I was struggling to balance emergency veterinary shifts and changing diapers, a friend asked me a simple question that I couldn't answer.

What's one of your favorite hobbies?

Seriously. I couldn't for the *life* of me answer this question. I mean, isn't cleaning a dirty nappy without getting poop on your hand a hobby? The hubster and I sort of treated changing diapers as an Olympic event!

Yet this question made me ponder a wee bit. It made me realize that since the Gillies were born, most of my hobbies had gotten pushed aside. Isn't that normal? Doesn't this happen to most folks? Seems like most of my reasons for why I couldn't do this or that was due to time, finances, or dare I say it, mama guilt!

Before the Gillies were born, I absolutely loved gardening, learning to play the guitar (only got to learning three chords), trail running, and pretending to be a food critic. I am not sure "pretending to be a food critic" could be considered a real hobby; however, it was one of my favorite recreational activities with friends. The criteria: you have to use ridiculous names, talk in fake accents, and order at least one appetizer, one entree, a side item, and a dessert to split! Pretty sure food critics don't behave this way, but we all have our things. At least I did—before the Gillies were born.

Now. I am not saying I am *not* grateful for the Gillies. I praise God for those littles every single day. It's just the last time I had a meal of my own without taking someone to the potty or cleaning up a snot rocket with my napkin was *ages* ago. Ah, memories.

So when my friend asked me this question and I stuttered to answer, I decided to talk it over with the hubster. Being parents didn't mean giving up on who we were; it was about *enhancing* who we were. Being parents no doubt made us better people. Since the Gillies were born, we have become stronger in our faith, become better communicators, got quite quirky and hilarious, plus developed a tolerance to answering 65,000 questions in one day. Yet we still needed to be *us* and find activities we not only enjoyed, but also could use to reduce stress.

Hobbies help you take a break. They help you expand your learning, develop new skills, and gain new wrinkles in your brain, like my hubster says. Other benefits include improving your mood and even creating positive social interactions. If you need help *choosing* a hobby, then let me share a fun little exercise and give you some examples.

How to find your hobby:

+ Set the timer on your alarm for five minutes.

+ Brainstorm all the things you love to do or have loved to do in the past. Anything counts!

+ Once the timer goes off, circle three hobbies that bring you the greatest joy.

+ Check your local area for classes, communities, church activities, clubs, etc. that host activities pertaining to one of the hobbies you circled.

+ Schedule time in your week for your new hobby.

+ Share your experience with your family at dinner. That's a bonus!

Some ideas for stress-reducing hobbies:

+ Get outdoors to hike, bike, run, bird-watch, tend a garden, paddleboard, etc.

+ Star gaze.

+ Explore the arts! Try painting, sculpting, visiting plays, joining a choir, or learning an instrument.

+ Learn how to knit or crochet.

+ Join a gym or take a boxing class.

+ Volunteer at the local community center.

Give Yourself A Break

The word "hustle" literally makes me cringe. People tend to think hustle is a good thing, but when I think of hustling, I think my emergency/critical care veterinary residency. I was working five to six days a week with 14- to 16-hour shifts. It felt at times I was surviving on a handful of hours of sleep and spending the rest of my time studying when not passed out on the floor. Now, granted, I signed up for my residency voluntarily and was extremely blessed to be a part of it. Plus, my resident mates, mentors, and the crew where I worked were phenomenal.

But, hustle makes me think of that period of my life because it was a wee bit out of balance, with lack of sleep and poor nutrition. Plus, if one stays out of balance for some time, the destination is most likely going to be *burnout*. No one needs imbalance and fatigue, especially when you are trying to hustle.

It's like a toddler on a sugar rush.... going... going... going... going... then BAM crashing hard. Drooling on yourself while you snooze from complete exhaustion. Did you get the visual?

To stay the course without the burnout and all the hustle, I'll share with you some of my favorite tips:

+ Work out: I aim for some sort of movement three to five days a week with rest days.

+ Sleep: Give your body time to rest (and digest) with at least seven hours of sleep.

+ Relationships: Unplug from the virtual space and be *present* with those you love.

+ Nature: Sometimes a dose of sunshine is what you need most.

Look at your planner and see—are you hustling a wee bit too much? Are you acting like a toddler on a sugar rush? When do you have time blocked to simply just *be*, and how are you going to give yourself a break today?

Make A "Ta-Da" List

"The key is not to prioritize what's on your schedule but to schedule your priorities." —Stephen Covey

Are you thinking, *duh*—schedule your life. Hello, that's nothing new.

Or maybe you're not a scheduler. Or you only schedule a few things, thinking, "I'll just remember [insert mundane task]." However, if we are being real here, if it's not on my schedule then it is 86 percent likely to get missed by me. So, I schedule it.

How exactly? Well. I simply take 20 minutes to look at my calendar for the next six days and write out my "TA-DAs" as I call them. The reason I call them "ta-da" is because it's a miracle when I get them all crossed off the list. So much so that I will actually say, *ta-da* as I cross it off my list. And ta-da sounds a lot less stressful than to-do.

{Plus. I love to cross things off my list; it's strangely satisfying... am I right?}

Here are the details with this one; they're quite simple. Schedule your life like a boss because you are the boss of your life, right? You are the leading lady in your own life! Hello, Kate Winslet movie reference. So schedule your non-negotiables and tasks you simply do not want to miss!

Things that help me with my ta-da list include the following:

+ Invest in a good planner. Some planners I love include Horacio planners, Passion Planner, and Corie Clark's Purposeful Planner.

+ Make a list of your non-negotiables: doctor's appointments, work meetings, date nights, after-school activities, hobby time.

+ Set the timer for 20 minutes and schedule your non-negotiables.

+ When the timer goes off, set it again for 10 minutes. Use this time to brainstorm your negotiables, meaning anything else you would like to make happen this week. Then prioritize this brain dump (i.e., what makes more sense this week: getting Fluffy a haircut or reorganizing the shoe closet?).

+ Once the timer goes off the second time, order your list of negotiables from 1 to 10 and put it in your calendar. If you have time this week to complete one or more of these tasks, fantastic! Cross them off the list. If not, no worries—they were negotiable, so move them to next week's list.

+ Just remember *you* are the leading lady in your life and boss of your schedule! Own it!

Become A Nap Ninja

This health hack is dedicated to my Grandma B, the original nap ninja. At 90 years old, she taught me the power of a good 15- to 20-minute power nap. Growing up, it was nothing for my grandparents to have family and friends over. It was also not uncommon for my grandma to disappear for 15 to 20 minutes while everyone was playing cards or taking a break for lunch.

By the time we realized she was gone, out popped her beautiful redhead into the room with a huge smile on her face. It wasn't until years later she confessed to me that she would go in the other room and take a 15-minute power nap on the floor behind the couch.

What the what?!?

Yes, my gorgeous ginger grandmother would be simply snoozing away—hidden from busy folks and catching up on her zzz's. The beautiful thing was, she came back refreshed and energized plus, no one knew. Genius.

Now, I'm not saying take a nap when company comes over. How rude? You have to understand when I was young, our family had epic card games that would last from mid-morning to the wee hours of the night. What I am stating is there is beauty in allowing your mind to drift off and giving your body's energy levels a chance to restore.

My favorite nap ninja tips:

+ Set your phone to DO NOT DISTURB (or airplane mode) and set an alarm for 15 minutes.

+ Lie down on the couch or bed and rest your eyes.

+ When the timer goes off, rise and shine. Move!

Move Your Tooshie

Sometimes, when I work it's like I'm in a trance—I completely zone out. It happened during vet school and throughout my residency. I could literally sit for hours lost in medical journals and books piled high with sticky notes scattered everywhere.

Now, with my focus switched a wee bit to *human* health (particularly the brain and gut), this trance-like state still exists. Just nowadays instead of reading about renal failure in dogs, I'm creating new recipes or writing blog posts about health hacks.

Yet here's the thing, love. Sitting your tooshie down for long periods of time isn't good for your health, your back, or your mind! During a Brendon Burchard conference, I learned we actually *lose* the ability to focus and be productive the longer we sit. Crazy, right?

This brings me to our final hack of this chapter: move your tooshie!! Here are some tips:

+ Simply set a timer on your phone for every 45 minutes. Please don't just make a mental note; you may not remember! The "Amber trance" exists for all of us.

+ When the timer goes off, just get up—stretch—move about the room—refill your water glass—take a five-minute dance break to a Meghan Trainor song {no judgey}. Just move! Get up and get your blood flowing. This will help revive those creative juices!

EVENING ROUTINE

I don't think I ever truly understood the value of a good night's rest until the Gillies came home from the NICU. Being born at 27 weeks, our twins were a wee bit tiny when we were finally able to bring them home. Due to their small size, we were told their feedings needed to occur every three hours. This meant the hubster and I were up for two hours at a time then slept for an hour to repeat over and over again. The first year with the Gillies home was such a blur of feedings, diaper changes, and snuggles. It's a time I loved and am extremely grateful for; however, my sleep suffered significantly.

It wasn't until the Gillies were around two years old that the hubster and I started researching how to get good quality sleep, seeing how the twins were *finally* (knock on wood) sleeping through the night, for the most part.

While reading books and listening to lectures on sleep, I realized that getting a good night's rest actually starts during the day! Yep, I said that right. In order for the hubster and I to get a good night's rest, we needed to prepare during the day—not just an hour before bedtime.

Now, the hubster and I have different sleep habits because, well, I'm currently not practicing veterinary medicine regularly. When I was working as an emergency veterinarian, my hours were all over the place with day shifts, swing shifts, and overnights. It was a mess for my circadian rhythm (a.k.a. sleep cycle). With the hubster's work, he is on call quite a bit, so his phone is always nearby and will ring in the middle of the night for emergencies.

So, this chapter is all about sharing some valuable tidbits that help me get a good night's sleep. Some hacks start during the day, and some lead up to the moment my head hits the pillow. The thing is, you do what's right for you, and if you are having trouble sleeping, don't hesitate to reach out to your primary care physician for medical advice.

Prep For Sleep During The Day

I remember participating in an ultimate frisbee competition in college. Seriously, it was amazing, and if I could find an adult version of ultimate frisbee near me, I would sign up in a heartbeat. Anywho, the day was filled with sunshine and endless rainbows while running around like a dog chasing a ball. By the end of the day, I was exhausted and fell into a deep slumber after a hot shower.

Why? Well, not just because I was tired from all the physical exertion. Most likely my ability to fall asleep easily had to do with getting enough sunlight *and* exercise, both of which help balance circadian rhythm.

Now, I'm not saying you have to sign up for flag football or join a cross-country team. If that's for you, fantastic. What I am saying is spending some time in the sunshine as well as breaking a sweat *may* help you rest better at night.

Here's how I prep my body for a good night's sleep during the day:

+   Spend time in the sunshine, especially first thing in the morning to help awaken the body and mind.

+   Get at least 20 minutes of physical exercise each day. This can look like a variety of activities such as going for a walk with the dogs, taking a yoga class, paddle boarding with a friend, pulling weeds in the garden, lifting weights or cycling, etc. Just move your body for 20 minutes.

Get Your Game Face On!

This health hack makes me chuckle because it sounds so silly; however, it's one of my favorite activities to do on Sunday evenings to prep my week for success. I *get my game face on* with a facial mask.

Ridiculous, right? I thought so as well, until I realized most bad-sassarinas do not take a beat for themselves—and that list once included *me*.

With homeschooling my twin six-year-olds, providing daily physical therapy for our sweet little man, coaching women on optimal wellness and business, and occasionally picking up relief shifts as a veterinarian, my self-care routine was being neglected.

So, I deemed Sundays FACE MASK day!

My favorite facial mask uses activated charcoal, which helps to draw out toxins and minimize my pores. Hello, yes and thank goodness. Now, whether you partake in face mask day or not is not the focus, love. The point is simply taking a beat to focus on self-care.

What is one self-care practice you have been putting off but would absolutely love to do? Something that brings you joy, makes you feel renewed, and may even restore a wee bit of "oomph" in your step?

For me, I prepare to *face* the week ahead by getting my *game face* on! Okay, those puns were really bad. I just had to, though. Your solution doesn't have to be facial masks; it can be anything that fills your cup. Other self-care practices could be: getting a manicure, listening to an audiobook, drawing a bath and soaking for a few minutes, meeting a friend for coffee, going for a long run, or even helping out a friend.

The point is—you do you, boo. However, if you are looking for a do-it-yourself facial mask recipe, here is one you can whip up in your kitchen and slather on tonight!

Do-It-Yourself Facial Mask Recipe

Ingredients

+ 2 tablespoons of pure honey
+ 1 teaspoon of cinnamon
+ 1 fresh lemon (use a wedge and squeeze out juice)

Now What?

1. Warm the honey for a few seconds, then sprinkle in the cinnamon as well as the juice from the lemon wedge.

2. Moisten (agh, I dislike that word)... *rinse* your face with warm water, then gently massage the mixture onto your face (avoid eyes) and allow to set for about 10 minutes.

3. Wash off with warm water and pat dry!

Hubster's Tip To Get Your ZZZ's

During my veterinary residency, my shifts were all over the place in regards to time of day. I would have a few day shifts in a row followed by a couple of swing shifts and then evening shifts. This meant my sleeping pattern was a wreck! It took me forever to get the hang of sleeping during the day; however, the hubster saved me with one amazing trick.

He bought me a silk eye mask that velcroed in the back. Genius!

Did you think I was going to say, he would turn down the thermostat to around 67 degrees Fahrenheit, which also helps you get a good night's sleep? Or were you thinking he removed all electronics from the bedroom so there were no blinking lights or distractions? That helps as well; however, the best sleep I got is when I used my amazing navy blue silk eye mask.

An eye mask will block out any light in the room, plus it can reduce noise if you purchase one that velcros in the back instead of using an elastic band. If you want to take this hack a step further, spritz a wee bit of lavender oil on the facial mask (on the outside, not the inside) and the calming scent will take you to dream land.

Turn Off Your Screens

This may be the hardest hack for most people—to simply reduce electronics at night time, well, at least an hour before bed!

Researchers even recommend removing the devices from your bedroom because the lights (blinking green lights indicating charging) can disrupt a good night's rest!

Without getting too science-y, here's the takeaway: Shutting down electronics at least an hour before bed gives your brain the ability to rest and sends the right signal that it's time for sleep.

One tip from me: Set your phone on Do Not Disturb at least thirty minutes before your bedtime, and make a habit of unplugging an hour before. Also consider adding a more relaxing habit, such as reading a good book, writing in a journal, or meditating.

Control Your Nightstand

One thing I have learned is the importance of gratitude and keeping your focus on the moments that bring you joy. Especially in today's world where we are constantly bombarded with social media, the news, and tons of other digital information, it is so easy to lose sight of life's joys, right? This is one of the reasons I keep a journal on my nightstand.

Journaling helps me refocus on what I am grateful for that day. In the morning, I will write down three things I'm grateful for, and in the evening I'll reread the list. The journal is also good for writing down tasks that were forgotten throughout the day, tasks that need to be done the next day, and any marvelous ideas that pop into my head throughout the night.

To be honest, the ideas that come to my mind at 2 a.m., which seem earth-shattering at the moment, are often complete nonsense—but at least I wrote them down!

Your journal doesn't have to be uber fancy; a college-ruled notebook will do just fine. The important thing is to keep a writing device (pen, pencil, plume) and some paper nearby so you can write down the top three things you are grateful for as well as any other ideas that may be swirling in your mind—so you can go to sleep with a grateful heart.

Add Some Green To Your Bedroom

Growing up, we used to say my mom had a certain green thumb—gangrene. This means my mom could bring a cactus or even a fake plant to a sudden death. It's like her superpower. One superpower, I am grateful to say, I did not acquire. If you have a thumb like my mom, this hack may not be for you; however, if you are up for a challenge, then consider adding some plants to your bedroom decor. Now, I am not saying to make your room resemble the rainforest; just one or two plants could help you get a better night's sleep.

You know that adequate sleep is crucial, but do you ever think of how air quality may be affecting your sleep? Plants are a cheap and effective way to improve the oxygen surrounding you and help you get a more peaceful sleep. A few plants I have stumbled upon that are good for the bedroom include English ivy, aloe vera plants, and the spider plant.

I hope you will incorporate some of these tips to help you get a good night's sleep. Need a recap?

+ Get out in nature first thing in the morning and soak up some sunshine.

+ Bust out a sweat for at least 20 minutes during the day.

+ Add some greenery to your bedroom.

+ An hour before you hit the sheets, unplug from electronics and turn down the thermostat to roughly 67 degrees Fahrenheit.

+ Take a beat for some self-care: facial mask, soak in the tub, read a good book, prioritize the spice cabinet, etc.

+ Place a journal on the nightstand and read the three things (from your morning routine) that bring you gratitude.

+ Spritz a wee bit of lavender oil on a silk eye mask and catch some zzz's.

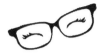

BE GOOD TO THE SKIN YOU'RE IN

It may be naive, but for the longest time I believed my skin would be absolutely flawless when I was mature, older… a mom. It's not like I had a horrible complexion. I think God balanced out the fact that I am super clumsy and quirky with a nice, even skin tone. However, I do occasionally get blackheads, especially when I have been studying for a bit, as I tend to rest my hands on my chin. I also get the monthly pimple that flares its nasty head during my Aunt Flow's visit… TMI? Probably.

But I actually believed my baby fine hair and the occasional pimple with blackheads would magically resolve when I was older. And yet, come to find out—I am quite mistaken. It seems my skin actually rebelled *after* I had the Gillies, and I found myself in my mid-thirties trying to learn more about *clean* beauty products and discovering a skin care routine that was right for me.

Now, I'm not going to share with you the products I use because let's face it (ha! pun not intended), what product works for me might not work for you. You have to discover that for yourself! Yet, what I will share with you are a few hacks I learned along my journey. Hacks that anyone can start doing to establish a cleaner, greener skin care routine.

Are you ready? Then buckle up, buttercup—this mama is going to share with you my favorite hacks for healthy skin!

What's On Your Pits?

Deodorant is one of those products that folks don't typically think about; it's simply a habit. And with each application, you get a wee bit of peace of mind that you won't stink up the place and/or you won't be sporting unpleasant sweat stains under your pits during this afternoon's office meeting. Right?

Well. In our journey towards a healthier lifestyle, I realized nutrition isn't the only thing that contributes to optimal brain and gut health, but other factors play a vital role as well. Things like your internal dialogue, daily habits, and even the products you place *on* your body.

The first place I started with our daily products was deodorant. Soon, I discovered there are at least *three* common ingredients found in conventional deodorants that scare me, but the main one is aluminum.

Aluminum is the primary ingredient in antiperspirant deodorants. It is a metal used to "block" the sweat glands. Questions have been raised recently about whether aluminum is related to serious medical conditions like Alzheimer's disease and breast cancer. We won't dive deep into the articles at this time; however, here are my thoughts. Why chance it? If a natural product works just as well as a product containing ingredients that scare me and could pose a health concern in the future, why not opt for the natural product?

Here are some tips for finding natural or "clean" beauty products:

+   Read the ingredients on the products you are using.

+   Research products and companies.

+   Find a product you love and a company you trust, then let me know!

Because the more you know, the more you can grow!

The Best Beauty Trick

A couple years back, I attended a mastermind retreat filled with brilliant women entrepreneurs. One of the ladies there knew my title as the Brain + Gut Health Explorer and how I strive to reduce toxins not only on my plate but also from our environment and products we use daily. She walked over to me and asked a simple question:

What is your best beauty trick for glowing skin?

The question caught me off guard and a lot of answers came to me all at once; however, one simple yet unglamorous hack stood out. Honestly, I think she assumed I would shout out a skin care line I love or some products I can't live without. Yet, her expression of complete shock and awe was priceless as I stated my answer.

Drink more water.

In a country where we have access to water all around us, I have heard the majority of Americans are chronically dehydrated. Yikes! Chronic dehydration doesn't just affect our moods but also our joints, digestive tracts, energy levels, and even our skin.

It's why this is one of my absolute favorite beauty tips: drink more water. A down-and-dirty trick is to drink half your body weight (pounds) in ounces throughout the day. This means a 140 lb woman would aim for at least 70 oz of water consumed throughout the day.

$$140 \text{ (lbs)} / 2 = 70 \text{ oz of water daily}$$

A few things I notice when I hit my water intake consistently is more energy, clearer skin, and less belly bloat. Can you say, sweet?!?

Here are a few tips that help me reach my water intake throughout the day:

+   Designate a water bottle just for you and keep it on hand all the time.

+   Wrap a rubber band along the bottom of the water bottle to remind yourself how many bottles' worth you need to drink throughout the day. When you refill your empty water bottle, simply remove one of the rubber bands to indicate how many times you need to refill your water bottle to reach your goal. (This tip is from my friend Kate!)

+   Before you drink a cup of coffee in the morning, drink 8 to 10 oz of water first.

+   When you wind down for the evening, drink 8 oz of water before hitting the sheets.

+   If you get hungry in the afternoon, drink a glass of water first. You might be confusing hunger with actual thirst!

Wash Your Face, Love

Most of us don't have a problem washing our faces at night, right? It's just a habit; however, folks may skimp out on a morning rinse-off. Why? Well, it's probably because you were just snoozing and thinking, *it's not like I was wearing makeup or ran a marathon. I was sleeping.*

But a lot happens while you sleep, love. Check it! Your body releases toxins, you may sweat a wee bit, and your pillowcases aren't 100 percent clean (especially if you live with pets).

So, if you have been skimping on rinsing your face in the morning, let this be a reminder to you to wash your face! Do not skimp out on it!

For me, I love rinsing off my face with cold water and applying a gentle moisturizer afterwards. The cold water definitely wakes me up, and I read once it helps slow the aging process as well as tighten your pores.

Is this true? I'm not completely sure, yet I do get questioned about my age quite a bit in the exam room with clients. One time, a client informed me he would rather answer my question when the doctor was present. The look on his face was priceless as I casually reminded him I was the veterinarian on staff that day.

Anywho, I also love to apply a gentle moisturizer with a wee bit of sunscreen. When applying, I use a jade roller to gently massage the product into my face as well as reduce any facial puffiness and increase lymphatic flow.

Need help remembering to wash your face? Simply set your washcloth underneath your toothbrush before going to bed. This way, when you head to the bathroom to brush your teeth in the morning, your washcloth will be ready as a gentle reminder to wash your face!

Protect The Skin You Are In!

A few years back, I spent time living in the West Indies. During the cold months here in the Pacific Northwest, I fantasize about those warm sunny days and the heat on my face. I remember on my very first weekend on the islands, I ran into another girl from the States at the local farmer's market.

I was dressed in a white t-shirt with cutoffs, which appeared to be my clothing staple, while she was decked out in the biggest floppy hat I had ever seen. Under the hat, she donned sunglasses with a full-sleeved rash guard and a sarong tied around her waist. There was no way any sunbeams were touching her.

It made me question my attire as well as how careless I was in regard to a serious situation: sun protection.

Nowadays with the Gillies, I'm vigilant about covering my kids head to toe in rash guards, floppy hats and sunscreen before we hit the pool or the park. Well, they don't wear rash guards at the park, but you get my gist.

And thanks to that encounter many years ago at a farmer's market in the

West Indies, I became aware and more educated about skin-sun protection, particularly with sunscreen. One of the things I look for in sunscreen is ingredients *not* included, such as parabens, fragrance, phthalates, and multiple ethoxylated ingredients. Plus, I like to opt out of anything in an aerosolized can!

Want to hear our tips on sun protection? Here goes:

+ Find shade: Picnic under a tree, take a canopy, or bring an umbrella. Staying in the shade could reduce your risk of burns.

+ Wear sunglasses: These are essential to help protect your eyes from UV radiation when you are in the sun all day long.

+ Wear clothes: Seriously, I learned this one from my friend at the West Indies farmer's market. Wear a rash guard or consider a shirt with sleeves, hat, shorts and/or cotton pants that are breathable. Stay cool and covered.

+ Play around the sun: This means go out when it isn't the hottest or the brightest.

+ Sunscreen: Um, obviously! Like I mentioned earlier, choose a sunscreen with the right ingredients—and wear it.

Take Care Of Your Feet

This will either make you laugh or you'll regurge a wee bit in your mouth. So brace yourself. Recently, I took our sweet little girl with me for a pedicure. We were celebrating how awesome she had been with traveling back and forth to physical therapy for her twin brother... when the lovely nail technician whipped out a freaking *cheese grater* on my feet. Yikes! I am not even joking.

A cheese grater.

This made me feel so much like a troll, but at the same time I knew my feet (especially my heels) had been neglected lately due to all of us running around and Mom not taking care of herself.

After the initial shock of horror washed over me, I was immediately filled with gratitude. Grateful to take a beat and protect my feet. It also made me think of ways I can take better care of my feet at home.

Here are some ways I tend to my feet—and why. Hopefully you can pick one or two tips to help you show your own feet some love.

+ Laying on my back with my legs up on a wall, I create a sort of "L" shape. This pose is quite relaxing and aids in blood circulation. It's especially helpful after a long day of sitting, either driving to physical therapy sessions or sitting at the desk writing this book.

+ Pedicure-spa day in our house! Once a week, the Gillies and I host a spa day where we break out towels, buckets of warm water, and pumice stones. We spend an hour soaking up our feet, spilling water everywhere, and lathering up lotion on our soles. You don't have to make such a huge mess like we do, but planning one day a week to soak your feet and lather them up will do wonders.

+ Each night, my feet get a gentle massage while I apply lotion, then I pull on wool socks. Yep, even in the hot summer months I like me some thick socks on my feet.

Consider Oil Pulling

Fun factoid: Each morning, I start with a dance session for at least ten minutes. Why do I do this? Besides pure bliss to dance first thing in the morning, it actually helps me not gag as the coconut oil pulling begins. My goal is to try oil pulling for at least twenty minutes, but I'm not quite there yet.

You most likely have heard of "oil pulling," which consists of swishing your mouth with coconut oil for about twenty minutes before spitting it out.

A few of the benefits folks have seen include whiter teeth, fresh breath, and antibacterial properties. Plus, some people even claim oil-pulling helps strengthen their gums and clear up their sinuses! What the what?!

Here's the thing—you do you, love! It may or may not be for you. Just do your research and choose what you think is best for *you*. I have read that oil pulling is an Ayurvedic method for detox and rejuvenation going back several thousand years.

Need to know my steps for starting with oil pulling? Here goes:

+ Brush your teeth as normal.

+ Using a tongue scraper, remove any excess debris from your tongue.

+ Floss to remove any debris from in between your teeth.

+ Take a teaspoon (some folks opt for more, but I like a teaspoon) of coconut oil and place in your mouth, then start swishing!

+ Turn on some music and dance it out as you swish in and out for approximately 10 to 20 minutes. I started with five minutes and gradually increased. Just do your best.

+ Do *not* swallow the coconut oil/saliva mixture. When finished, spit it into a cup or trash can. You do not want to spit in the sink, because once coconut oil cools, it will solidify and could possibly clog your drain. Not good!

+ Gargle with a mixture of sea salt and warm water, then spit it out.

+ Brush your teeth once more without toothpaste to clean off any stubborn particles that remain. And you are done!

Be Sweet To Your Skin

Earlier, we talked briefly about skin and sun protection, but let's dive a wee bit more into how we can be even sweeter to our skin. See, our skin is the largest and fastest growing organ we have. Isn't that crazy!?

Your skin protects you from a plethora of harmful threats every single day. {Let's be real, I just wanted to use the word "plethora."} One way I care for mine is by using an all-natural body scrub, which you can easily whip up in your kitchen.

Sugar Scrub Recipe

Ingredients

+ 1 cup of sugar
+ 1 cup of frozen blueberries
+ ½ cup of coconut oil (room temperature)
+ Few drops of lavender essential oil

Now What?

Blueberries are known to be loaded with antioxidants, which is great for the skin, and sugar is an excellent exfoliator. I also like to add a wee bit of lavender essential oil to give my scrub a relaxing, spa-like vibe.

Now simply take a gallon Ziploc® bag and place the blueberries in it. Seal the bag. Crush the blueberries with a rolling pin on top of the bag. In a bowl, combine the sugar with the crushed blueberries. Once combined, stir in the oils. Place the mixture into a sealed glass container and keep it airtight. I like to use mine within a week!

To use, apply a small amount on your wet skin and scrub gently. Rinse off and pat dry. Avoid contact with open wounds, eyes, or any sensitive areas. As always, be careful in the bathtub. Use caution so you don't slip and hurt yourself!

Making myself a DIY body scrub is one of my favorite ways to be "sweet to my skin." Another idea is scheduling yourself a deep tissue massage! Am I right?

Let's recap how to be good to the skin you're in:

+ Read the ingredients on the products you are using.

+ Research products and companies; find a product you love and a company you trust.

+ Hydrate yourself properly with fresh, clean water.

+ Protect your skin from the sun with good shades, proper attire, playing around the sun's hardest rays, and sunscreen.

+ Be kind to your skin and feet.

+ Consider oil pulling.

+ And love, wash your face!

TRANSFORM YOUR BODY AND MIND WITH MOVEMENT

When you hear the word *transformation*, what comes to mind? Some people think about a weight loss journey while others may think about a mindset shift. Well, for me, I get an image of a butterfly emerging from a cocoon filled with battle scars, memories of the obstacles overcome, and a beautiful new beginning.

It's also how I view my own transformation, my own journey—which, when I look at the entire picture, is the epitome of a hot mess. Literally. And I am in love with it.

See. It's not just about the pounds I lost, but about the strength I have gained both physically and mentally. It's about mental toughness and how the relationship I developed with God became stronger. It's about the *people* who rallied with me and those who picked me up, lent me support, provided me with a roof over my head or a kind word in the darkness. It's about the knowledge I learned and, most importantly, the truth I have found about myself.

For instance. I have overcome my obsession with counting calories and developed a healthy relationship with food. I've been a size 16 and a size 2, as well as all the sizes in between. I've been able to lift 100 pounds and not even lift myself out of bed on hard days. I've been able to run 150 miles and incapable of running *one*. I've been in a dark place where I felt like nothing I did was right, yet I've also been content with the person I turned out to be.

Transformations make pretty pictures, but the journey—the *process* of the transformation—is not so pretty. It's not bright and shiny. It's not full of smiles and sunshine. The process can be discouraging at times, and you've got to develop perseverance—as well as realize your vision goes beyond what you're tempted to settle for. The ugly process of transformation involves facing your fears, pushing past them, and *using* them to fuel your fire.

Transformations are not simple, yet the process as a whole is rather remarkable. I hope no matter your end goal, you use your fear, the doubt, the dark times, and allow them to propel you forward and transform you into the person you want to be. Yet, remember to be gentle with yourself throughout the process.

This chapter along with the next is centered on my own transformation story—both the physical (fitness) and mental aspects. I'll share with you some of my favorite hacks that helped me *move* my tooshie and be the mom the Gillies needed me to be.

See, our son needs his mom right now to lift him and sometimes carry him distances while still keeping an eye on his sister. My body needs to be strong and full of energy for my children. It doesn't need to be free of cellulite, which I call thigh dimples because my body is so happy! And my body doesn't need to be rocking a six pack. Now, would I be happy if my body did both of those things—um, yes. But I am more happy my body is able to catch my twins when we are playing tag in the yard and dance with the hubster in the kitchen when no one is looking.

These are my hacks for fitness, but this is *your* journey and your transformation.

Find A Workout You Love

Most of us know all the benefits of breaking a consistent sweat through exercise. These include improved mood, better sleep, reduced stress—the list goes on. Yet some of us, past-me included, may think workouts need to be intense to be good, and that's not the case.

Workouts can be *anything*, love. Nowadays, a variety of workouts are available through different mediums—gym classes, rock climbing, barre classes, hot yoga, crossfit box sessions, roller skating outside, workout videos you can do at home, cycling inside or outdoors, etc.

One thing I learned is my workout does not have to look like yours, hers, or even his—yet it should be something that produces a good sweat, and bonus points if it's fun.

So here's my question to you. What do you like to do for movement? Just find a good workout that you find FUN because you'll be more likely to work out consistently! And as always, check with your primary care physician before starting any new workout regimen, okay? Okay.

Need some ideas on what type of exercises and programs are out there, well, I've got you covered. Here are a few:

+ Check your local area for any crossfit boxes near you and take an introduction class to see if you like it.

+ Are you more into cycling? Join a local cycle group, take a spin class, or invest in a Peloton® bike and cycle at home!

+ Interested in yoga? Check YouTube for some classes online, sign up for a monthly membership at a local yoga studio, or look into virtual yoga programs.

+ More into the outdoors, are you? Well. Lace up and go for a walk around the neighborhood with your dog, consider taking a rock-climbing class or joining the nearby community rowing club.

No matter what it is, find something that's enjoyable to you and move your body. My goal is 20 to 30 minutes of movement each day for increased energy, a happier mood, and mental clarity!

Schedule Movement Like A Boss

You ever hear something that sounds completely ridiculous, yet when you follow through with it, you realize it's pure genius? Well, this hack is just like that. *Learn to schedule exercise like an appointment.* If you think of exercise like a meeting with *you*, the CEO of your body, you would be less likely to skip out on the meeting, right? Right!

Whether you are just starting out or an exercise pro, all it takes is a few moments once a week to jot down exactly when and where you are going to work out, along with noting any equipment needed.

For me, every Sunday afternoon, I take a glance at my weekly schedule and write out the non-negotiables. You guessed it, workouts are a non-negotiable! Remember, I am the CEO of my overall wellness, so I need to schedule these "meetings."

Now, I get it—life happens. Sometimes, the Gillies wake up before I'm ready or through with my workout. You know what, that's okay! The point is, I get 100 percent more workouts in if I *schedule* them on my planner than when I just wing it.

Here are my tips for scheduling your workouts:

+ Remember, you are the boss of your overall wellness. Stop canceling appointments with yourself and get moving, no matter how slow!

+ Choose a few days a week for exercise, and be realistic when setting the times. If you aren't an early bird but schedule your workouts before sunrise, you most likely will be hitting snooze instead of crushing those workouts.

+ Look at the whole picture of your week. Is there time to schedule a walk during lunch break? Would your best friend consider going to a yoga class instead of meeting up for drinks after work on Wednesday? Your workout schedule doesn't have to look like mine or even be pretty; it just needs to happen.

Work Out Even On Vacation

One thing I tell my clients is not to go more than two days in a row without exercise. This may not sound challenging, except it applies to vacation days, too! When on vacation, it is so easy to get caught up in the simple act of relaxation and exploring the local cuisine. Now, I'm not saying don't relax and have fun on vacation. What I *am* saying is simply think about ways to explore your current environment with movement.

Options could include going paddle boarding, renting a bike to tour the town, walking the streets after dinner, visiting the museums or zoos, or even taking a fitness class that's not offered back home (you may even score a free visitor pass to the gym)!

You never know what's out there, so get out and explore the area. Plus, when you get back from vacation, you will feel more refreshed and energized to get back into your normal routine.

Up Your Workout Attire

There seriously may be some underlying psychological reasoning behind this, but when I wear amazing workout attire, I feel inspired, and it literally gives me an energy boost! So, for anyone who loves to shop, I'm giving you a reason to ditch the uncomfortable workout clothes and snag some new ones!

You don't have to buy expensive exercise clothes to get a good workout, but there's evidence to suggest that clothes might actually play a role in keeping you motivated during a workout. For a long time, I would just wear what-ever clothes I had lying around, which included an extra-large Tweety Bird T-shirt that would get heavy with sweat, and I would waste time to roll up my sleeves every few minutes. It was ridiculous, especially since I've learned that wearing uncomfortable clothes might be what stands between you and a good workout.

When you are planning your workouts, take a beat to evaluate what you will be wearing. Give yourself permission to toss any clothes that do not inspire you or could cause any unnecessary chafing or discomfort. Find clothes that motivate you and make you feel confident! Again, they don't have to be expensive. For instance, I snagged my favorite leggings on Amazon for less than twenty dollars, and they have outlasted others purchased from some pretty top-dollar companies.

Need some ideas for shopping for workout attire? Here goes:

+ Check out off-season deals at your local stores or outlet malls. This may mean you purchase your swimsuit in the fall or winter jacket in the summer.

+ Be aware of online deals, and stock up on your favorite items!

Invest In Workout Socks

The other day, I asked the hubster to grab me a pair of socks on his way back from the bedroom because I wanted to head out for a run. Oh, my lanta! He came back with a pair of knee-length argyle socks.

Let us all pause for effect.

Can you just imagine me running down the road wearing my ninja-style black running pants with brown and navy argyle socks stitched together with yellow thread? Insert: sexy ninja nerd alert.

At this moment, I realize some folks may not understand the importance of workout socks! Before I go on, I will ease your mind and let you know I did run outside with my argyle socks. And I did so with confidence. Now, socks are basically an extension of your shoe and protect your feet from the impact as well as the conditions your feet will endure during a workout.

Choosing a sock that provides cushion, wicks away the sweat, and doesn't slip is crucial for an effective workout. A good pair of socks will also prevent you from obtaining blisters. Invest in high quality socks and wear them solely for workouts. Please do not let them be your everyday socks and definitely not knee-length blue and brown argyle socks with yellow stitching.

Here are a few of my favorite workout socks. Remember to check your local stores for deals:

+ Injinji Toe Socks

+ Smartwool PhD

+ Thorlos Experia No-Show Performance

+ Balega Hidden Comfort No-Show Running

Set Out Your Clothes

I played basketball in high school, and practice was held in the early morning before class. The night before, I would pack my gym bag with clothes to wear for school. That way when my alarm went off, all I had to do was switch into my gym clothes, grab my bag and go! The main reason I did this was to sleep as long as possible, but it also helped reduce any early morning decision making.

I still benefit from this habit today. I don't pack a gym bag anymore (our gym is the garage), but I still lay out my clothes the night before and even took it a step further by reducing my wardrobe to only white T-shirts and green scrub pants.

That's right folks, just call me a fashionista! And yes, I'm living dangerously in those white T-shirts with twins in the house.

The point is not that you have to wear something simple or the same thing every day. (Although this is a habit adopted by some brilliant creators.) The simple task of laying out your clothes the night before like you were taught in grade school *may* help your mornings run a tad bit smoother and reduce some decisions you have to make before your first sip of coffee.

There are no additional hacks for this one; just simply leave your clothes out the night before and *voila*, you've mastered this hack!

Link Arms With A Fitness Buddy

Back in college, I found my very first fitness buddy. She also happened to be my college roommate who was amazing in so many ways—one of which was pushing me out the door for our morning walks on days when I was dragging my feet. We would walk for an hour or less around campus soaking in the morning sun and just catching up on what was happening in our lives. It was magical to break a sweat and connect with a friend. By the time I got back to our dorm room, it felt like *anything* was possible that day.

Now, you may have an accountability partner for certain life goals or your business, which is fantastic. However, I recommend you also have someone in your corner specifically to offer support when you are trying to reach a health or fitness goal.

There is a trick, though, to selecting a fitness buddy. It's one you may not have thought about, so lean in and let me tell you. *Reach out to someone with whom who you are friendly but not necessarily close.* If you must choose your spouse, though, make sure neither of you takes things too personally or gets competitive, because the plan could go south.

My best friends and the hubster are not my fitness accountability partners, ever. Why, exactly?

Well, the hubster has a background playing college football and powerlifting, so he can get a wee competitive. As for as my best friends, they will usually allow me to bail on my workouts because they just want me to be happy. Plus, they tend to not want to give me the tough love I need when I drag my feet or give them a lame excuse as to why I don't want to work out that day.

It also happens that my best friends usually do not have the same fitness goals I do, which is okay. One of my goals is to be known as an ultra-trail marathoner, while my friend finds complete joy in aerial yoga. This means she may not fully understand why I need to bust my tooshie with sprints on a Tuesday. That's fine; it's not her job to fully understand.

Here's the thing, though. You need to evaluate your personal goals in regard to your own health and fitness. This is where the fun begins with exploring classes nearby, online programs, or local accountability groups. Then link arms with someone who has similar fitness goals as you and whose personality meshes well with yours. Find someone who will cheer you on but at the same time, will not let you bail because of your lame excuse.

This takes trial and error, but when you find this person, do not let her go! And remember to always cheer your buddy on and push her towards her goals as well.

Mix Up Your Workout Routine

Earlier we mentioned the benefits of working out: gain more energy, get better quality sleep, handle stress effectively, burn fat, strengthen bones, boost your brain, regular poopage (TMI?). Plus, in my opinion, the best type of workout for you is the one that gets you moving and inspired. Some folks love water aerobics while others love karate or barre classes or boxing.

However, if you are looking to kick your fitness routine up a notch, then switch things up! This will create muscle confusion (a good thing), help your brain stay sharp, and keep you from hitting a plateau. For me, weekly workouts include a mix of high-intensity interval training (HIIT), sprints, weights, and flexibility. This allows my body time to rest, recover, strengthen, and build endurance.

Here are some tips to help you think outside the box for mixing up your routine without straying too far:

+ If you enjoy walking/running: roller skating, ice skating, hiking, or cycling

+ If you enjoy being in/on the water: water aerobics, paddle boarding, swimming, or paddle board yoga classes

+ If you enjoy crossfit: boxing classes, hot yoga, or steel mace workouts

+ If you enjoy yoga: paddle board yoga classes (obviously, I want to try this), aerial yoga, or pole dancing classes

Active Recovery

When I hit a plateau with my fitness goals, I reached out to a dear friend who happens to be a phenomenal fitness trainer. She had me discuss in great detail the struggles I was facing as well as my nutrition and workout plan.

With a deep sigh, she informed me of her recommendation—which took me by surprise. Her expert advice was to rest just a day or two a week in what she called *active recovery*.

Now, active recovery is just a fancy way of saying "give your body some time to rest, but don't just lounge on the couch binge-watching Netflix and eating Cheetos." Although, the latter option sounds a wee bit good right about now, am I right?

The first few weeks definitely felt strange as I refrained from going for a run or breaking out the weights. However, my body responded quite well, and some of the benefits I noticed included faster recovery, more endurance, and a happier gut.

Some ways you can add active recovery into your week is by going for a leisurely walk with a friend or your pup, joining in on a yoga class, hitting the pool for a swim, or chasing toddlers around the park. On second thought, scratch that last one. Chasing the twins around the park is anything but recovering.

The key is to simply take time to move a wee bit less intensely once or twice a week and see the amazing things your body can do the next time you are ready to crush a workout.

Add Some Foam Rolling

A dear friend once told me, "Foam rolling is a poor man's massage." Now, being a twin mom who absolutely loves deep tissue massages yet doesn't actually have the time or a local place to snag one, this sounded like a win. I invested in a foam roller, which is freaking bru- to the -tal, but also quite amazing.

Every Sunday evening, I take a beat to brew a pot of white pomegranate tea, which I enjoy sipping while wearing my activated charcoal mask and doing 20 minutes of foam rolling. Can you just picture this? Isn't my hubster a blessed man!

When I first started foam rolling, I had no idea what I was doing and in fact did everything wrong. I purchased a foam roller that wasn't smooth but had knobs. Don't do that if you're just starting out. I also would roll the foam roller over parts of my calves and thighs quickly. Don't do that, either. The point is to roll slowly over your muscles to allow the tense areas to relax.

I carry most of my tension in my calves, and I will spend every second of those 20 minutes foam rolling my calves. It may be because I'm a runner or the fact that I chase twins all day. My former life as an emergency veterinarian may have something to do with it, also. All I know is, foam rolling feels amazing if you do it correctly and consistently.

Foam rolling offers tons of benefits such as improving range of motion, relaxing muscles, and aiding in recovery. But I'll remind you foam rolling *may not* feel great to you. I know, I am not selling it. Just wanted to warn you, though.

Here are some of my tips for foam rolling:

+ Purchase a *smooth* foam roller rather than one with knobs all over the place.

+ Try to relax while foam rolling because when you tense up, you will not be able to get down into those knotted areas. Hubster calls these areas "trigger points."

+ Never roll on a joint, bone, or your lower back. Just no.

+ Go slowly over your muscles. (I like to do my calves and thighs.) When you find one of your "trigger points," go back over the area slowly and even hold on that spot for a bit.

+ Focus on your breathing, as this will help you relax while you roll.

+ If you're a visual learner, check out YouTube for foam rolling videos! This was where I learned the basics of foam rolling.

+ Always when starting something new, discuss it with your primary care physician and get the go-ahead before foam rolling for the first time.

Fuel Your Body Well Post Workout

In order to know *what* to eat and *when*, we need to listen to our bodies. What works for me may not exactly be the thing for you, and that's okay. I just want to fill you in on how I fuel my body and why.

I typically skip breakfast and work out on a "fasted" gut, because it makes my body freaking rejoice. For years, I have tried to be the type of person whose body enjoyed breakfast; however, after a few vomit episodes in grade school, I realized my body does not like breakfast.

Do not get me wrong—I love a hearty breakfast filled with droopy eggs and leafy greens; however, my timing for breakfast is pushed back a few hours to around eleven, which makes my body so much happier.

So because I work out in the mornings before breakfast, my body is in a "fasted" state during exercise. This is said to help speed metabolism, build muscle, and increase energy levels. All I know is my body prefers it. Some folks need to have a quick meal before working out, and that's great. You do what's right for you and your body. Basically, listen to your gut.

But now let's talk about fueling your body right *after* a workout.

This can be a wee bit tricky because if you are like me, you are hungry yet you don't want to screw up all your hard work, right? You want to make sure you are fueling your body with foods it needs.

After a workout, my body needs good protein, healthy fats, and complex carbohydrates. Did your eyes roll for a second? I apologize, let's take a beat to create what a plate would like for me after a workout.

First, start with complex carbohydrates. Your body burns through glycogen (for energy) while you are working out. So, you want complex carbs afterwards because they are easy to digest and will replace the lost glycogen. My go-to is sweet potatoes!

I love them mashed up, diced and roasted, placed in a spiralizer for noodles, or chopped into bits in a food processor then sauteed for couple of minutes as a substitute for rice. Sweet potato "rice" is so good.

The second item to consider is protein. Your muscles need fuel to help repair. Pasture-raised eggs are a favorite of mine. Here's the thing about eggs—and this can definitely be a soapbox for me, so I'll keep it short. How the chickens are raised along with the diet the chickens are fed affects the quality of yolks. When you can, purchase your eggs locally from a nearby farm, and try to get in the habit of reading labels. What I look for on the label is "pasture-raised" chickens, and I *avoid* words such as "vegetarian diet" or "grain diet."

The third item I add to my plate is a healthy fat, which for me includes avocado because it's known as "God's butter" and has amazing benefits such as an excellent source of potassium and fiber! Other healthy fat options include coconut oil, walnuts, almonds, tuna, and salmon.

Now to top off my plate, I throw in some leafy greens. Who says leafy greens can't be for breakfast, right? Spinach, kale, arugula, asparagus, and sometimes Brussels sprouts make the cut. We have been taught since grade school that eating leafy greens is good for our health, so why not start adding them to the first meal of your day?

With my plate crafted, you can see my favorite go-to post-workout meal is typically sunny side up eggs over sweet potato noodles with sauteed greens and a side of avocado. Oh, so good. If that doesn't sound completely delicious to you, then consider having:

+ A superfood smoothie: blended vegan protein powder, leafy greens, avocado, almond milk (the avocado in the smoothie actually gives a creamy texture)

+ A bowl of oatmeal with almond butter and blueberries on top, then save the greens for a salad at lunch.

Here are a few things to consider:

+ Does your body respond better working out in a fasted or non-fasted state?

+ When do you typically break your fast? The majority of folks "fast" overnight during sleep. How long is your fast, and what time do you break it with "break-fast"?

+ Have a plan for what to eat *after* your workout, and do not just whip something up when you are in a hangry state. Poor choices get made then.

+ Create your top three favorite "go-to" post-workout recipes so you have something to gravitate toward in a pinch!

YOUR BIGGEST WEAPON IS WITHIN YOU

Back in college, I worked in a local bookstore, which was completely fabulous. It was dimly lit and smelled like dusty paperback books, with fresh coffee brewed and local baked goods on display. Light jazz music played gently in the background, and if you came in the afternoon, you could catch a glimpse of the two slightly obese cats snoozing in the window display. Each day I went to work was like walking onto a movie set of a romantic comedy, with potential for a "meet cue" with my love interest. I loved every minute of it.

Besides the owner of the shop, there was another worker who was slightly older and so much cooler than me. We each had a section of the store we fancied, and mine—if you could guess it—was the chick-lit section. This was the section filled with books on, well, female heroines and romantic comedies. Oh, my Doris Day-Debbie Reynolds loving heart.

One section I never took the time to browse was the self-help aisle, which is quite hilarious as the majority of my bookshelves nowadays are filled with personal development books. In college, I had not yet uncovered the powerful tool I possess. A tool we all possess. One that can help us change our course of action. One that can help us conquer impossible feats.

The tool I'm referring to is our mind.

Ugh, if I could go back and talk to my younger self, I would tell her to stop being such a twit and go in the self-help aisle to start feeding her mind with powerful, inspiring messages.

See, what you feed your mind matters, and I'm not just talking about books.

Your mind is taking in messages all around you from the people you hang out with, your social media feed, the news you are watching, and even the habits you are forming. Your brain is soaking it all in, love.

So, I'm going to share with you some of my favorite personal development hacks to help you strengthen your biggest weapon—your mind.

Celebrate Others

The Gillies are the masterminds of this hack. Every day, they take a moment to tell me how "awesome" I am doing—with little hand fist-bumps, stickers, and even "well, that's awesome, Mama" shouts throughout the day. They are seriously going to give me a big head, but I've heard adolescence is when they'll deflate the ego. Guess I'll take all the celebrations I can get even if it's just because I put the dishes in the dishwasher. Yes, they even tell me "good job" for putting up the dishes! Oh my heart.

Here's the thing. It is so easy to get caught up in the day-to-day and focus so much on our own struggles, that we miss opportunities to celebrate others. Yet celebrating others is one thing that can definitely fill *your* cup and give another person a boost, too!

It doesn't have to be much. Check it, a "good job with the dishes, Mama" makes my heart swell! Just take a beat to think about folks you encounter throughout the day. Who can you give a shout-out to today? Need some ideas, here you go:

+ Make a list of all the folks you engage with in a day. Choose one person a day to give a compliment or positive word. You can do this in person, with a sticky note on their desk, or even a voice text!

+ If you spend much of your time on social media, consider starting your day with gratitude before you get into the "scroll zone." Choose one friend who is on your mind and send her or him a quick message just sharing how much you appreciate that person as a friend.

Laugh Hard And Laugh Often

I came across a quote from Maya Angelou that said, "Laugh as much as possible, always laugh. It's the sweetest thing one can do for oneself and one's fellow human beings."

Isn't that beautiful? Laughing is one of my favorite pastimes. I'll fill you in on a little story: growing up I honestly thought I was God's comic relief. This is not a joke. Whenever something was troubling in the world, God would take a glance at my life and simply chuckle at the ridiculousness of what I was doing. Why? Well, I know I'm a wee bit quirky. This isn't some secret; it is quite obvious, and when I was little, it was my greatest gift.

You might recall from chapter one that I am the youngest of three girls. My two older sisters were confined to wheelchairs when I was young, due to a genetic condition. I made it my job to get my sisters to laugh each day. And laugh hard—you know, the deep belly laughs that cause you to snort and almost tinkle on yourself.

I took this job quite seriously growing up. I would pretend the bathtub was a race car and act out driving in the Indy 500, only to crash into theatrics on the bathroom floor. Next, the kitchen would turn into the Olympic stage as I attempted unsuccessfully to slide across the floor and flip, using the cabinets and refrigerator door handle to hoist myself into the air. This is something I wouldn't recommend. The fireplace would turn into a tightrope in a circus as I hummed my own theme music while my sisters would chuckle at my silliness. Still today, when I visit, it's my main goal to get my sister laughing and laughing hard.

Laughing has some amazing benefits, such as reducing cortisol (the stress hormone), increasing pain tolerance, breeding resilience, and improving mood. I am pretty sure you knew the last one, you smart cookie.

With this hack, I just want you to take a beat to laugh. I know sometimes we get in a dark place and it can be extremely difficult to find anything enjoyable. Friend, I understand. If you are in that place, please find a friend to talk to, and surround yourself with a loving environment. I'll share some of my favorite ways to enjoy a laugh:

+ Meet up with a friend and just hang out. No agenda.

+ Rent a comedy and spend a couple of hours just focused on the laughs.

+ Ask your grandparents to tell you a joke. Some of my best jokes come from my PawPaw.

+ Catch a live comedy act in your local area.

+ Go to the nearest bookstore or library and pick up a clean joke book for kids. It's hilarious how ridiculous some of those jokes can be.

+ Snag a few laugh taffys. I'm serious.

Give Thanks

This hack will be short and simple, yet sometimes those are the most powerful messages. We are *all* on a journey, whether it's with business, relationships, health, fitness, mindset. Each one of us is moving on this journey and facing obstacles along the way.

Yet we also come across individuals who help us, either with words of encouragement, guidance, or just emotional support. I bet if you took a beat right now, a person may pop into your mind who has helped you over the course of your journey.

Well, this hack is to simply say, "thank you." Thank you to the person who was a light along your way. Thank you to the person who lifted you up when you were struggling. Thank you to the person who didn't judge you or ask questions, but just supported you. Thank you to the person who shared a kind word at just the right moment.

It's so easy to get caught up in our journey, focused on the obstacles and the "to-do" list we set for ourselves. This also makes it easy to forget those who help us along the way. Form a monthly habit of reflection and gratitude. Here's how:

+ Each month, reflect on what you accomplished, and list anyone who helped you in any way to make those accomplishments happen.

+ If you can, send a handwritten letter to each person just thanking them and expressing your appreciation in words. I know it's easier to send a direct message on social media or shoot an email, yet there's something powerful in receiving a written word of thanks.

Lean In And Toss Out Perfection

Have you ever started a habit, but life derailed you from your goal? Then instead of picking up the pieces from where you left off, you completely gave up. Yes, it is all right. You can raise your hand, too. I have done this numerous times, but here's the thing.

Perfection does not exist, love.

Striving for perfection usually leads to disaster and worse yet, *inaction*! No matter if you are talking about relationships, business, or fitness goals—toss out perfection and lean in to the process.

Lean in to the uncomfortable.

Lean in to the conversations.

Lean in to the experience.

Lean in to the journey.

Sometimes you just need to take a deep breath and fully embrace what's in front of you. This reminds me of a time I had to fully lean in and release the idea of perfection. It was about a year ago; I was sitting in a room filled with inspiring women entrepreneurs. In my mind, I had what I thought was the perfect plan for my business. While I sat there, listening to our host speak words I did not want to hear, I realized her words were truth. The words made me face a wall I had placed around myself. The words forced me to see things I just didn't want to see.

Instead of leaning in to the truth, I resisted. I felt fear of the uncertain, of the uncomfortable, and of how this truth didn't fit into what I thought was my perfect business plan. Yet, after wiping my tears, I leaned in and gained so much clarity. It was like a lightbulb finally clicked, and the dimly lit place where I stood opened a path illuminated before me. Isn't it amazing what you can learn when you take a breath, allow yourself to lean in, and release the idea of perfection?

Stay Present

Saying this makes me feel so old, but in today's world it feels like something is always competing for our attention. The news, podcasts, social media, marketing ads, emails, notifications on our phones, and new apps coming out each day. There is always something happening and fighting to be seen. When I brought this up to my grandparents, their comment was so simple. "Amber, there has always been something happening in the world. And the world keeps turning."

Those words shook me because I am blessed my grandparents are getting closer each day to turning 93 years old. During their time, they have seen some iconic moments, and they are right—the world kept turning.

Yet how can I reduce the distractions from our lives and be fully in the moment? If there has always been something happening in the world and now I'm more acutely aware of it due to technology, what action steps can I take to stay present? This was on my mind right before the hubster and I relocated our family cross-country. We took a gander at the items we wanted to bring with us on our new adventure as well as the habits we wanted to instill in our family.

Now, you don't need a cross-country move to do this, or even a fresh New Year start. You don't need the first of the month or even a Monday. You just have to take a beat, write your list, and take action. I'll be honest though, clearing the slate before our family's cross-country move was much needed. As a person who loves to make lists, the 32-hour road trip to our new home was the perfect time to brainstorm healthy habits our family can develop to ensure we're staying present with one another.

Here's our list, and I hope it will inspire you to create your own!

+ Unplugged family dinners each night. No technology at the table except for the hubster's phone when he is on-call, yet it has to be off the table and within earshot.

+ Saturday morning outings to the local farmer's market and grocery shopping. I love involving the Gillies in the grocery shopping, even though it can be a wee bit of a hassle. They are more inclined to eat the meals I cook because they are aware of the goodness of the ingredients and how the whole process works from farm to table. Plus, they each get to pick out *one* snack for the week ahead.

+ Sunday church service, whether in real life or virtual sermon. Just praising God each Sunday morning and having a discussion afterwards fills my heart.

+ Start the day with morning prayers and meditation as well as movement. The Gillies always remind me when I do not say our affirmations and meditations. It's beautiful to see how they find joy in these daily habits as well.

+ Weather permitting, go outside in nature for at least 10 to 20 minutes each day!

+ Take a beat at the end of the day to say one thing we are grateful for and one thing we completely failed at doing. Why do I like to talk about failure? To show the Gillies failure isn't a bad thing; it simply means you did not accomplish your end goal—yet there is always a lesson learned. Plus, the most important thing is that they tried!

+ Each parent has a "date" with each kid individually each month, and bonus points if Mom and Dad venture out of the house for a date once a month, too.

Protect Your Inner Circle

You've most likely heard the saying, "You are the sum of the five folks you hang around the most," which I'm obviously paraphrasing. This does scare me a wee bit since 40 percent of my five people are six-year-olds. I'm just chalking this up to mean I can explain numerous things at a kindergarten level while simultaneously cooking a meal and wiping snot from a child's face.

Back to the quote—you should protect your inner circle. Your inner circle is the folks you spend the most time with, love. Here's the thing, when you are around folks who are inspiring, positive, and focused on a mission, it is their words that will inspire you. Their dreams, visions, and habits will sink in and affect how you think, how you work, and the habits you form.

This is why most business folks do best in a mastermind group. It is why having a fitness group or partner for accountability allows people to crush their health goals. Because you are all inspiring one another toward a like-minded goal. It may not be exactly the same goal, but together you encourage one another to move forward.

Take a glimpse of the folks with whom you spend the majority of your time. As I mentioned earlier, two of the five people in my inner circle are the Gillies, our six-year-old twins. But seriously, if the members of your inner circle are not goal-driven or do not speak positivity, then maybe it's time to protect your inner circle and gradually put space between yourself and others.

I know that was extremely tough to hear, and I realize you may have some folks in your life that you cannot completely ignore or push out. I'm not saying you should. What I am saying is, protect who *you* choose to spend your days with and surround yourself with. Choose people who lift you up, motivate you, and inspire you to take action toward your goals.

So what about the folks surrounding you who do not inspire you, like a coworker, for instance? Let me share with you this tip I learned along my journey. It started as a joke between the hubster and me, then turned into something I actually do. There was a particular person I had to encounter, yet every time I was around that person, my skin would crawl and I could sense my energy levels changing. I joked to the hubster how I needed to put up my "happy shield" so I could reflect her negative energy (insert laser beam sounds here).

Over time, this evolved into imagining myself putting on a jacket and literally zipping it up. Doing this gave me peace knowing that even though I had to encounter this person, I was able to protect my energy, my goals, and my inspirations.

Sometimes to protect your inner circle, you may find yourself zipping up your metaphorical jacket or putting up your happy shield. No matter what you choose, just remember to be kind to the other person as well as yourself, and protect your inner circle.

Flip Your Script, Friend

Anyone can change their behavior, their habits, and accomplish their dreams, but it all starts with your mindset. This hack is all about flipping the negative chatter you whisper to yourself into a more positive statement in order to watch the universe unfold its goodness.

Here is a simple yet powerful hack I learned while reading one of Jen Sincero's books. Take a beat to think of one thing you are constantly mumbling to yourself. It may be, "I am not professional enough to go live on social media." Oh, wait. That's something I used to mumble to myself. But, let's use that one as an example.

If you are constantly mumbling something to yourself that is a wee bit negative, your voice and the words you speak to yourself are the ones your mind constantly hears. If you continue to speak these words to yourself, where do you think you will be in a year or even five years from now? Most likely in the same place, mumbling the same words to yourself.

Instead I challenge you to take your "saying" and flip the verbiage to a more positive statement. Rather than saying, "I am not professional enough to go live on social media," I would flip to a more positive meaning such as, "The people I am serving appreciate my authenticity and real life vibe when I go live on social media."

How much more powerful is that statement? Again, I challenge you to zero in on the main message you are mumbling to yourself—the one that hinders you from taking action towards your dream. Then play around with the words so you can flip the switch to a powerful and positive statement.

Stop Flaking On You, Love

Yesterday, you said tomorrow.

Ouch, right? This was the conversation I had with myself one morning, as I laced up my shoes and headed out for some trail running. For a bit, it seemed like I kept putting off going for a run, which is sad because running outdoors fills my cup. That is when it hit me—I keep flaking on myself!

You know what I am talking about, right? When you tell your friend you are up for the party happening this weekend, but then Friday comes around, and you just want to cuddle up on the couch to binge-watch your favorite season on Netflix. That is called flaking. The majority of us have done it at some point in our lives.

Yet each time I postpone my hair appointment or bail on the hot yoga class, it's more than just "flaking." What I am really saying to myself is, "There's something more important than me and my health at this moment."

Oh, that hurts. Especially when I wonder, what is more important than my health? Without my health, I cannot take care of the Gillies. Without my health, I cannot coach my clients. Without my health, I cannot shower my hubster with love or support my friends.

How can I take care of anyone or anything if I am not taking care of me? How can you, love? Let that sink in for a few moments. I'll wait . . . .

Today I am giving myself as well as you permission to stop flaking on ourselves and do something to take care of us! This doesn't have to be huge, like booking a yoga retreat with your girlfriends in Bali—which sounds absolutely sublime—but it does have to be something that fills you.

Here are some ideas to help you brainstorm ways to take care of you:

+   Book yourself that massage you have been desperately needing, even if it's just a foot massage. It's magic.

+   Go for an afternoon stroll or lace up those shoes for a quick run on the trails.

+   Schedule an appointment with yourself for a matinee movie, and enjoy watching it solo.

+   Take an Epsom salt bath with some light music playing, and dim the lights. Just be careful getting out of the tub because you will be so relaxed.

+   Consider a hobby in gardening, playing a new instrument, taking a hip-hop class, or painting pottery.

Speak Kindly To Yourself

Let's get a wee bit real, love. We have been through a lot together in this book, I mean I shared embarrassing stories of my childhood and how I watch YouTube videos while on the toilet. So, why not share this as well?

The phrase "self-love" is one I had trouble fully grasping. See, it's one thing to love how your body responds and its capability to move. But, it's another thing to love your body's appearance. Am I right? The combination, I am convinced, is the beauty of self-love.

This doesn't mean you aren't trying to improve your appearance or your body's capabilities; it just means you love where you are and appreciate the journey of where you are headed. And you love all the bits of it. Even the wobbly ones.

Self-love is a practice I am currently working on, and my journey to fully love all aspects of myself began when I was informed one of the babies inside my pregnant belly was a girl. Why did that matter? Well, I knew if our son had my hubster's genes, he would absolutely love his body. That is a trait of my hubster's I just admire—his ability to love every single bit of his body. Ugh, why does he have this superpower but I don't? Enough whining, Amber.

I knew with our little girl, I wanted her to fall in love with all of her body and appreciate everything her body was able to do. Yet in order for this to happen, I needed to set the example and start loving myself and all the wobbly bits. Or in my case, crooked bits.

See. For the longest time, I refused to look at myself in pictures. I would literally cringe when I'd see a photo of myself smiling because my front tooth is slightly crooked. I used to have perfectly straight teeth until a head-butting incident, paired with my refusal to fully commit to wearing a retainer, came into play! I became so aware of this crooked tooth that smiling in public happened only when part of my face was hidden, my teeth weren't showing, or I was captured at a certain angle.

Can you imagine how exhausting that was? It took a lot of digging deep to realize I was the only one who saw my tooth this way, and the hubster even digs it! I was definitely the only one wasting good energy worrying about it. After some time, I have learned to love the crooked right tooth. It actually goes quite nicely with my slightly quirky personality. Yet this love didn't happen overnight.

Here are some things that helped me "love" my crooked bits and maybe will help you, too:

+ List all the amazing things your body is capable of doing. Yes, I mean all. We all have talents, and it's time we write them down to see it. Some folks can sing. Some folks can paint like Bob Ross. Some folks can dance in a car and make it resemble a seizing cat. We all have talents. Write yours down.

+ Take a beat to look in the mirror and write down all the things you love about your body. Your shoulders and how amazing they look in tank tops. How those black leggings make your tooshie look firm.

+ Is there one area you are refusing to look at? Why, exactly? Be honest with yourself. For me, it was my crooked tooth and my smile. Write all the things you LOVE about this area you are refusing to look at. For instance, I love how my smile makes my nose crinkle. I love how my smile radiates to my eyes and they sparkle. I love how my sister and I have the same crooked tooth—and I love her smile!

+ Now, write on a sticky note and tack to your mirror a list of all the things you love about your body part you are refusing to look at. And each day, thank yourself for this body part. Remind yourself what you love about this body part. Remind yourself to show it off!

+ Remember you are beautifully and wonderfully made—all the bits of you. Self-love, to me, is all about appreciating what your body can do and loving your body now, as is.

Face Your Wall

On the day of our tenth wedding anniversary, I faced my wall. We all have a wall, which surrounds us in our comfortable, cozy life bubble. It's a boundary that could hinder us from reaching our goals, setting new limits, and pushing us further.

Well, allow me to fill you in on my wall. A few years back, the hubster and I decided to celebrate our 10th wedding anniversary by participating in a Spartan race. The fact that we came out of the race alive, still speaking and married, makes me quite relieved. I signed us up, so naturally, we did not participate in the shortest race with the least amount of obstacles. Why would I sign us up for that one? {Insert: sarcasm.} Because I still feel like we are in college in the prime of our athletic ability.

I remember the morning of the race like it was yesterday. We headed out before sunrise to drive five hours to the event and even stopped at a hole-in-the-wall gas station to get breakfast burritos (hello, *huge* mistake). We talked about the obstacles and what we expected as well as what we feared.

While the hubster was more nervous about the running distance, I was terrified of hurling myself over a 6- to 7-foot wall. This makes sense since I'm 5'4" with a three inch vertical.

We got to the event, parked and walked to the starting line—when I saw it. MY WALL. The thing I was most afraid of was staring right at me. In order to get to the starting line, you had to cross over a 6- to 7-foot wall. YIKES! Did you catch that? I'll repeat it for you.

BEFORE you got to the starting point, you would have to throw yourself over a WALL.

It was at this point, I just started laughing—because the main thing I was scared of could hinder me from getting to the start line!

Spoiler alert: I made it over the wall in one piece and through the other obstacles—AROO!

There was one thought that kept popping up in my mind as we ran the course. *We all have walls.* Walls we set up to protect ourselves, but over time these walls can actually *hinder* us from our greatest potential!

Here are some tips to help you face your wall:

+ Take a beat to think about what walls you may be setting up around you. Is that wall serving to protect you or hinder you from your start line?

+ Write down three to five action steps you can take to scale your wall.

+ Next, choose a deadline for each action step and write it down. Deadlines should be doable yet not overwhelming. Also, do not set them so far in advance that you may lose focus. I like to set 90-day goals with monthly action steps because I can break down those action steps into smaller weekly goals. You do you, boo.

+ Finally, tell a friend about your action steps and your goal. Fill her in on the deadline you choose for each action step and give her permission to hold you accountable.

Be You, Love

Here's the last hack and quite possibly my favorite tip in this chapter. It's one I uncovered once I became a mom, and it's so simple.

Be you.

That's it! I discovered it while reading a bedtime story to the Gillies one night.

Seriously, have you ever noticed that children's books are basically self-help or personal development books for little kids? This fascinates me. I didn't realize it until I was in the midst of reading to our twins when *BAM* a simple one-liner in the book became a life lesson for this mom.

Dr. Seuss told me, "Be who YOU ARE and say what you feel, because those who mind don't matter and those who matter don't mind."

Life lesson, right? Be you!

It's something I have to remind myself daily because with technology nowa-days, we have access to enter into anyone's life and see their highlight reel on social media at any moment. With this capability, it is also quite easy to start leaning towards comparing yourself and your life to what you are seeing on social media. This cannot be healthy.

A friend of mine calls it "comparitis."

Comparitis (noun): an inflamed condition that is inflicted because you compare yourself to someone else. That's my medical talk for you and it's complete hogwash, but the meaning is there.

Looking at yourself, your journey, or the moment you are currently in, and comparing it to something you visualize on social media or even in a brief moment in real life is unhealthy. In a photo you see a mere glimpse of what's happening. You don't see the trials a person went through, the obstacles they have overcome, or how many filters they have had to use. You just see a snapshot. That's it.

Now, I'm not just preaching to you. I am preaching to myself because it is so easy to catch "comparitis" and forget the simple children's book mantra, Be You. So, here are some of my favorite hacks for getting rid of comparitis:

+ Find things you enjoy doing—and do them.

+ Unplug from technology for a couple hours a day and be fully present in life.

+ Reduce the time you set to scroll on social media. Consider taking a social media detox every month for a few days.

+ If you have to unfollow folks whom you notice yourself "comparing to," then do it. Follow folks who inspire you instead.

+ Read children's books out loud and often. Consider volunteering to read at a local bookstore, library, or school.

+ Watch a Disney movie. I am not even playing with this one. Something about watching a Disney movie and seeing the heroine fight for her truth just gives me warm fuzzies. My favorites are *Moana* and *Mulan*.

FINAL WORDS

As I stated in the beginning of this book, this "No-Brainer" journey for me started out because I forgot who I was after the birth of our twins. If I am being completely honest with myself, I probably forgot who she was even before we were pregnant. By focusing on becoming just one percent better each day, I fell in love with taking care of me and discovered who I was. It wasn't about a certain jean size, even though putting on jeans seems like the trigger for me. There was so much happening behind the scenes; the bedazzled jeans were just a catalyst for this journey.

And it's a journey I am grateful to still be on and to be able to share with you. This book is filled with some of my favorite hacks, which helped me reduce the dreaded brain fog, gain clean energy and stop reaching for an afternoon latte, plus increase my productivity. How else do you think I'm able to homeschool the twins, provide physical therapy to our little man, coach clients with their business, and write this book? This mom needs all the energy and all the hacks.

But there's just one little thing I want to share with you. When considering all the information you've just read in this book, I would love for you to feel like it's just a friend sharing her favorite secrets with you. You listen, maybe laugh here and nod your head there—but please don't think you have to do them all. You don't. Pick one you think will help you and try it out for a while, like your favorite pair of bedazzled jeans.

While on this journey of aiming for one percent better, just remember to not lose focus on the good stuff. And that includes you, love. How about one more story before we wrap things up, shall we?

Picture this: It was a warm sunny day in the Texas heat. For some ungodly known reason, I decided to take my afternoon workout outside. My outfit of choice was going to be running pants and a tank top but the hubster casually mentioned, "It's 90 degrees outside and you may want to consider shorts, love."

Smart man.

Now, it should be noted that I rarely wear shorts because of paleness, thigh dimples (we call it thigh laugh lines, most folks call it cellulite), and varicose veins. I'm a work in progress, too.

Yet this time, I thought, "why not?" We were currently living in the boonies where no one could possibly see me, and there was the benefit of getting some vitamin D on these legs. After digging in the closet for my only pair of workout shorts, I pulled them up quickly and raced into the living room to head outside.

While racing out the door, I passed in front of the twins and our little man looked up to say,

"Mama, you are wearing shorts. You are gorgeous!"

Ugh, you guessed it—waterworks.

I broke out crying right there because as you've probably figured out by now, I am a major weeper. We hugged for a brief moment as I mumbled "thank you," and I walked outside to start the workout.

During my run, my son's words kept playing in my mind—*you are gorgeous*! Each time I glanced down and attempted to look at my legs (difficult when the paleness is blinding you with the sun), I heard his words.

This experience made me realize two things:

1. Our twins don't see Mama's cellulite, I mean thigh dimples. They don't see Mama's pale legs. They don't see Mama's varicose veins. They don't see Mama's patchy hair job. They simply see their mama.

2. I am obviously *not* 100 percent happy with my legs' appearance, but I do see all the good my legs do for me. I truly appreciate their ability to walk, to chase after the Gillies in the living room, to dance with them in the kitchen, to carry Little Man when he needs me, etc. I am in awe of their strength to constantly lift things and to run—heck, they carried my booty 150 miles across the Sahara desert. These legs are amazing and quite beautiful! And every day, I strive to make them one percent better with walking, foam rolling, lifting, dancing, etc.

And this is what I want you to notice, whether it's your thighs or your crooked smile or even your lack of energy in the afternoon. There is goodness in you. I believe it's truly okay *not* to be completely happy about a situation, but do not focus on the negative. Continue to do better, to BE better, even if it's just one percent each day. Because, friend, you are worth it, and taking care of you should be a *no-brainer*!

FURTHER BOOK RECOMMENDATIONS

+ *Body Love* by Kelly LeVeque (Harper Collins, 2017)

+ *131 Method* by Chalene Johnson (Hay House Inc., 2019)

+ *Tools of Titans* by Tim Ferris (Houghton Mifflin Harcourt, 2016)

+ *Discipline Equals Freedom* by Jocko Willink (St. Martin's Press, 2017)

+ *High Performance Habits* by Brendon Burchard (Hay House Inc., 2017)

+ *The 5 Second Rule* by Mel Robbins (A Savio Republic Book, 2017)

+ *The Compound Effect* by Darren Hardy (Da Capo Press, 2013)

+ *You are a Badass* by Jen Sincero (Running Press, 2013)

+ *It Starts with Food* by Dallas and Melissa Hartwig (Victory Belt Publishing Inc, 2012)

+ *The Better Brain Solution* by Steven Masley, M.D. (Alfred A. Knopf, 2018)

+ *Girl, Wash Your Face* by Rachel Hollis (Nelson Books, 2018)

+ *Shut Up and Run* by Robin Arzon (Harper Design, 2016)

ABOUT THE AUTHOR

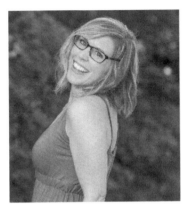

Amber Langley Gill, DVM, is a former emergency/critical care veterinarian who stepped away from the clinical floor and into the role of Brain + Gut Health Explorer. After the premature birth of her twins, whom she calls the Gillies, Amber's main priority was understanding the brain-gut connection and simple health hacks she could implement for her children's well-being. She now coaches women and fellow mompreneurs through the journey of physical and mental wellness. Amber resides in northern Idaho with her wonderfully supportive husband, the Gillies, and multiple family pets. This is her first book.

Made in the USA
Middletown, DE
11 December 2019